American Psychiatric Association
1400 K Street, N.W., Washington, DC 20005
www.psych.org

ISSN 1067-8743
ISBN 0-89042-319-9

CONTENTS

Visit **www.psych.org**
for Continuing Medical Education credit and
Quick Reference Guides for this and other APA Practice Guidelines.

STATEMENT OF INTENT

This report is not intended to be construed or to serve as a standard of medical care. Standards of medical care are determined on the basis of all clinical data available for an individual case and are subject to change as scientific knowledge and technology advance and patterns evolve. These parameters of practice should be considered guidelines only. Adherence to them will not ensure a successful outcome in every case, nor should they be construed as including all proper methods of care or excluding other acceptable methods of care aimed at the same results. The ultimate judgment regarding a particular clinical procedure or treatment plan must be made by the psychiatrist in light of the clinical data presented by the patient and the diagnostic and treatment options available.

This practice guideline has been developed by psychiatrists who are in active clinical practice. In addition, some contributors are primarily involved in research or other academic endeavors. It is possible that through such activities some contributors have received income related to treatments discussed in this guideline. A number of mechanisms are in place to minimize the potential for producing biased recommendations due to conflicts of interest. The guideline has been extensively reviewed by members of APA as well as by representatives from related fields. Contributors and reviewers have all been asked to base their recommendations on an objective evaluation of available evidence. Any contributor or reviewer who has a potential conflict of interest that may bias (or appear to bias) his or her work has been asked to notify the APA Department of Quality Improvement and Psychiatric Services. This potential bias is then discussed with the work group chair and the chair of the Steering Committee on Practice Guidelines. Further action depends on the assessment of the potential bias.

This practice guideline was approved in July 2001 and published in October 2001.

GUIDE TO USING THIS PRACTICE GUIDELINE

This practice guideline offers treatment recommendations based on available evidence and clinical consensus to help psychiatrists develop plans for the care of adult patients with borderline personality disorder. This guideline contains many sections, not all of which will be equally useful for all readers. The following guide is designed to help readers find the sections that will be most useful to them.

Part A contains the treatment recommendations for patients with borderline personality disorder. Section I is the summary of treatment recommendations, which includes the main treatment recommendations along with codes that indicate the degree of clinical confidence in each recommendation. Section II is a guide to the formulation and implementation of a treatment plan for the individual patient. This section includes all of the treatment recommendations. Section III, "Special Features Influencing Treatment," discusses a range of clinical considerations that could alter the general recommendations discussed in Section II. Section IV addresses risk management issues that should be considered when treating patients with borderline personality disorder.

Part B, "Background Information and Review of Available Evidence," presents, in detail, the evidence underlying the treatment recommendations of Part A. Section V provides an overview of DSM-IV-TR criteria, prevalence rates for borderline personality disorder, and general information on its natural history and course. Section VI is a structured review and synthesis of published literature regarding the available treatments for borderline personality disorder.

Part C, "Future Research Needs," draws from the previous sections to summarize those areas in which better research data are needed to guide clinical decisions.

INTRODUCTION

This practice guideline summarizes data regarding the care of patients with borderline personality disorder.

Borderline personality disorder is the most common personality disorder in clinical settings, and it is present in cultures around the world. However, this disorder is often incorrectly diagnosed or underdiagnosed in clinical practice. Borderline personality disorder causes marked distress and impairment in social, occupational, and role functioning, and it is associated with high rates of self-destructive behavior (e.g., suicide attempts) and completed suicide.

The essential feature of borderline personality disorder is a pervasive pattern of instability of interpersonal relationships, affects, and self-image, as well as marked impulsivity. These characteristics begin by early adulthood and are present in a variety of contexts. The diagnostic criteria are shown in Table 1. For the diagnosis to be given, five of nine criteria must be present. The polythetic nature of the criteria set reflects the heterogeneity of the disorder. The core features of borderline personality disorder can also be conceptualized as consisting of a number of psychopathological dimensions (e.g., impulsivity, affective instability). A more complete description of the disorder, including its clinical features, assessment, differential diagnosis, epidemiology, and natural history and course, is provided in Part B of this guideline.

This guideline reviews the treatment that patients with borderline personality disorder may need. Psychiatrists care for patients in many different settings and serve a variety of functions and thus should either provide or recommend the appropriate treatment for patients with borderline personality disorder. In addition, many patients have comorbid conditions that may need treatment. Therefore, psychiatrists caring for patients with borderline personality disorder should consider, but not be limited to, treatments recommended in this guideline.

TABLE 1. Diagnostic Criteria for Borderline Personality Disorder[a]

A pervasive pattern of instability of interpersonal relationships, self-image, and affects, and marked impulsivity beginning by early adulthood and present in a variety of contexts, as indicated by five (or more) of the following:

(1) Frantic efforts to avoid real or imagined abandonment[b]
(2) A pattern of unstable and intense interpersonal relationships characterized by alternating between extremes of idealization and devaluation
(3) Identity disturbance: markedly and persistently unstable self-image or sense of self
(4) Impulsivity in at least two areas that are potentially self-damaging (e.g., spending, sex, substance abuse, reckless driving, binge eating)[b]
(5) Recurrent suicidal behavior, gestures, or threats, or self-mutilating behavior
(6) Affective instability due to a marked reactivity of mood (e.g., intense episodic dysphoria, irritability, or anxiety usually lasting a few hours and only rarely more than a few days)
(7) Chronic feelings of emptiness
(8) Inappropriate, intense anger or difficulty controlling anger (e.g., frequent displays of temper, constant anger, recurrent physical fights)
(9) Transient, stress-related paranoid ideation or severe dissociative symptoms

[a]From DSM-IV-TR (1).
[b]Excluding suicidal or self-mutilating behavior (covered in criterion 5).

OVERVIEW OF GUIDELINE DEVELOPMENT PROCESS

This document is a practical guide to the management of patients—primarily adults over the age of 18—with borderline personality disorder and represents a synthesis of current scientific knowledge and rational clinical practice. This guideline strives to be as free as possible of bias toward any theoretical approach to treatment.

This practice guideline was developed under the auspices of the Steering Committee on Practice Guidelines. The process is detailed in a document available from the APA Department of Quality Improvement and Psychiatric Services: the "APA Guideline Development Process." Key features of the process include the following:

- A comprehensive literature review and development of evidence tables.
- Initial drafting by a work group that included psychiatrists with clinical and research expertise in borderline personality disorder.
- The production of multiple drafts with widespread review, in which 13 organizations and more than 60 individuals submitted significant comments.
- Approval by the APA Assembly and Board of Trustees.
- Planned revisions at regular intervals.

A computerized search of the relevant literature from MEDLINE and PsycINFO was conducted.

The first literature search was conducted by searching MEDLINE for the period from 1966 to December 1998 and used the key words "borderline personality disorder," "therapy," "drug therapy," "psychotherapy," "pharmacotherapy," "psychopharmacology," "group psychotherapy," "hysteroid dysphoria," "parasuicidal," "emotionally unstable," and "treatment." A total of 1,562 citations were found.

The literature search conducted by using PsycINFO covered the period from 1967 to November 1998 and used the key words "borderline personality disorder," "hysteroid dysphoria," "parasuicidal," "emotionally unstable," "therapy," "treatment," "psychopharmacology," "pharmacotherapy," "borderline states," "cognitive therapy," "drug therapy," "electroconvulsive shock therapy," "family therapy," "group therapy," "insulin shock therapy," "milieu therapy," "occupational therapy," "psychoanalysis," and "somatic treatment." A total of 2,460 citations were found.

An additional literature search was conducted by using MEDLINE for the period from 1990 to 1999 and the key words "self mutilation" and "mental retardation." A total of 182 citations were found.

Additional, less formal literature searches were conducted by APA staff and individual members of the work group on borderline personality disorder.

The recommendations are based on the best available data and clinical consensus. The summary of treatment recommendations is keyed according to the level of confidence with which each recommendation is made. In addition, each reference is followed by a letter code in brackets that indicates the nature of the supporting evidence.

PART A:
TREATMENT RECOMMENDATIONS FOR PATIENTS WITH BORDERLINE PERSONALITY DISORDER

I. EXECUTIVE SUMMARY OF RECOMMENDATIONS

A. CODING SYSTEM

Each recommendation is identified as falling into one of three categories of endorsement, indicated by a bracketed Roman numeral following the statement. The three categories represent varying levels of clinical confidence regarding the recommendation:

I. Recommended with substantial clinical confidence.
II. Recommended with moderate clinical confidence.
III. May be recommended on the basis of individual circumstances.

B. GENERAL CONSIDERATIONS

Borderline personality disorder is the most common personality disorder in clinical settings. It is characterized by marked distress and functional impairment, and it is associated with high rates of self-destructive behavior (e.g., suicide attempts) and completed suicide. The care of patients with borderline personality disorder involves a comprehensive array of approaches. This guideline presents treatment options and addresses factors that need to be considered when treating a patient with borderline personality disorder.

C. SUMMARY OF RECOMMENDATIONS

1. The initial assessment

The psychiatrist first performs an initial assessment of the patient to determine the treatment setting [I]. Because suicidal ideation and suicide attempts are common, safety issues should be given priority, and a thorough safety evaluation should be done. This evaluation, as well as consideration of other clinical factors, will determine the necessary treatment setting (e.g., outpatient or inpatient). A more comprehensive evaluation of the patient should then be completed [I]. It is important at the outset of treatment to establish a clear and explicit treatment framework [I], which includes establishing agreement with the patient about the treatment goals.

2. Psychiatric management

Psychiatric management forms the foundation of treatment for all patients. The primary treatment for borderline personality disorder is psychotherapy, complemented by symptom-targeted pharmacotherapy [I]. In addition, psychiatric management consists of a broad array of ongoing activities and interventions that should be instituted by the psychiatrist for all patients with borderline personality disorder [I]. Regardless of the specific primary and adjunctive treatment modalities selected, it is important to continue providing psychiatric management throughout the course of treatment. The components of psychiatric management for patients with borderline personality disorder include responding to crises and monitoring the patient's safety, establishing and maintaining a therapeutic framework and alliance, providing education about borderline personality disorder and its treatment, coordinating treatment provided by multiple clinicians, monitoring the patient's progress, and reassessing the effectiveness of the treatment plan. The psychiatrist must also be aware of and manage potential problems involving splitting (see section II.B.6.a.) and boundaries (see section II.B.6.b.).

3. Principles of treatment selection

a) Type.   Certain types of psychotherapy (as well as other psychosocial modalities) and certain psychotropic medications are effective in the treatment of borderline personality disorder [I]. Although it has not been empirically established that one approach is more effective than another, clinical experience suggests that most patients with borderline personality disorder will need extended psychotherapy to attain and maintain lasting improvement in their personality, interpersonal problems, and overall functioning [II]. Pharmacotherapy often has an important adjunctive role, especially for diminution of symptoms such as affective instability, impulsivity, psychotic-like symptoms, and self-destructive behavior [I]. No studies have compared a combination of psychotherapy and pharmacotherapy to either treatment alone, but clinical experience indicates that many patients will benefit most from a combination of these treatments [II].

b) Focus.   Treatment planning should address borderline personality disorder as well as comorbid axis I and axis II disorders, with priority established according to risk or predominant symptoms [I].

c) Flexibility.   Because comorbid disorders are often present and each patient's history is unique, and because of the heterogeneous nature of borderline personality disorder, the treatment plan needs to be flexible, adapted to the needs of the individual patient [I]. Flexibility is also needed to respond to the changing characteristics of patients over time.

d) Role of patient preference.   Treatment should be a collaborative process between patient and clinician(s), and patient preference is an important factor to consider when developing an individual treatment plan [I].

e) Multiple- versus single-clinician treatment.   Treatment by a single clinician and treatment by more than one clinician are both viable approaches [II]. Treatment by multiple clinicians has potential advantages but may become fragmented; good collaboration among treatment team members and clarity of roles are essential [I].

4. Specific treatment strategies

a) Psychotherapy. Two psychotherapeutic approaches have been shown in randomized controlled trials to have efficacy: psychoanalytic/psychodynamic therapy and dialectical behavior therapy [I]. The treatment provided in these trials has three key features: weekly meetings with an individual therapist, one or more weekly group sessions, and meetings of therapists for consultation/supervision. No results are available from direct comparisons of these two approaches to suggest which patients may respond better to which type of treatment. Although brief therapy for borderline personality disorder has not been systematically examined, studies of more extended treatment suggest that substantial improvement may not occur until after approximately 1 year of psychotherapeutic intervention has been provided; many patients require even longer treatment.

Clinical experience suggests that there are a number of common features that help guide the psychotherapist, regardless of the specific type of therapy used [I]. These features include building a strong therapeutic alliance and monitoring self-destructive and suicidal behaviors. Some therapists create a hierarchy of priorities to consider in the treatment (e.g., first focusing on suicidal behavior). Other valuable interventions include validating the patient's suffering and experience as well as helping the patient take responsibility for his or her actions. Because patients with borderline personality disorder may exhibit a broad array of strengths and weaknesses, flexibility is a crucial aspect of effective therapy. Other components of effective therapy for patients with borderline personality disorder include managing feelings (in both patient and therapist), promoting reflection rather than impulsive action, diminishing the patient's tendency to engage in splitting, and setting limits on any self-destructive behaviors.

Individual psychodynamic psychotherapy without concomitant group therapy or other partial hospital modalities has some empirical support [II]. The literature on group therapy or group skills training for patients with borderline personality disorder is limited but indicates that this treatment may be helpful [II]. Group approaches are usually used in combination with individual therapy and other types of treatment. The published literature on couples therapy is limited but suggests that it may be a useful and, at times, essential adjunctive treatment modality. However, it is not recommended as the only form of treatment for patients with borderline personality disorder [II]. While data on family therapy are also limited, they suggest that a psychoeducational approach may be beneficial [II]. Published clinical reports differ in their recommendations about the appropriateness of family therapy and family involvement in the treatment; family therapy is not recommended as the only form of treatment for patients with borderline personality disorder [II].

b) Pharmacotherapy and other somatic treatment. Pharmacotherapy is used to treat state symptoms during periods of acute decompensation as well as trait vulnerabilities. Symptoms exhibited by patients with borderline personality disorder often fall within three behavioral dimensions—affective dysregulation, impulsive-behavioral dyscontrol, and cognitive-perceptual difficulties—for which specific pharmacological treatment strategies can be used.

i) Treatment of affective dysregulation symptoms. Patients with borderline personality disorder displaying this dimension exhibit mood lability, rejection sensitivity, inappropriate intense anger, depressive "mood crashes," or outbursts of temper. These symptoms should be treated initially with a selective serotonin reuptake inhibitor (SSRI) or related antidepressant such as venlafaxine [I]. Studies of tricyclic anti-depressants have produced inconsistent results. When affective dysregulation appears as anxiety, treatment with an SSRI may be insufficient, and addition of a benzodiazepine should be considered, although research on these medications in patients with borderline personality disorder is limited, and their use carries some potential risk [III].

When affective dysregulation appears as disinhibited anger that coexists with other affective symptoms, SSRIs are also the treatment of choice [II]. Clinical experience suggests that for patients with severe behavioral dyscontrol, low-dose neuroleptics can be added to the regimen for rapid response and improvement of affective symptoms [II].

Although the efficacy of monoamine oxidase inhibitors (MAOIs) for affective dysregulation in patients with borderline personality disorder has strong empirical support, MAOIs are not a first-line treatment because of the risk of serious side effects and the difficulties with adherence to required dietary restrictions [I]. Mood stabilizers (lithium, valproate, carbamazepine) are another second-line (or adjunctive) treatment for affective dysregulation, although studies of these approaches are limited [II]. There is a paucity of data on the efficacy of ECT for treatment of affective dysregulation symptoms in patients with borderline personality disorder. Clinical experience suggests that while ECT may sometimes be indicated for patients with comorbid severe axis I depression that is resistant to pharmacotherapy, affective features of borderline personality disorder are unlikely to respond to ECT [II].

An algorithm depicting steps that can be taken in treating symptoms of affective dysregulation in patients with borderline personality disorder is shown in Appendix 1.

ii) Treatment of impulsive-behavioral dyscontrol symptoms. Patients with borderline personality disorder displaying this dimension exhibit impulsive aggression, self-mutilation, or self-damaging behavior (e.g., promiscuous sex, substance abuse, reckless spending). As seen in Appendix 2, SSRIs are the initial treatment of choice [I]. When behavioral dyscontrol poses a serious threat to the patient's safety, it may be necessary to add a low-dose neuroleptic to the SSRI [II]. Clinical experience suggests that partial efficacy of an SSRI may be enhanced by adding lithium [II]. If an SSRI is ineffective, switching to an MAOI may be considered [II]. Use of valproate or carbamazepine may also be considered for impulse control, although there are few studies of these treatments for impulsive aggression in patients with borderline personality disorder [II]. Preliminary evidence suggests that atypical neuroleptics may have some efficacy for impulsivity in patients with borderline personality disorder [II].

iii) Treatment of cognitive-perceptual symptoms. Patients with borderline personality disorder displaying this dimension exhibit suspiciousness, referential thinking, paranoid ideation, illusions, derealization, depersonalization, or hallucination-like symptoms. As seen in Appendix 3, low-dose neuroleptics are the treatment of choice for these symptoms [I]. These medications may improve not only psychotic-like symptoms but also depressed mood, impulsivity, and anger/hostility. If response is suboptimal, the dose should be increased to a range suitable for treating axis I disorders [II].

5. Special features influencing treatment

Treatment planning and implementation should reflect consideration of the following characteristics: comorbidity with axis I and other axis II disorders, problematic substance use, violent behavior and antisocial traits, chronic self-destructive behavior, trauma and posttraumatic stress disorder (PTSD), dissociative features, psychosocial stressors, gender, age, and cultural factors [I].

6. Risk management issues

Attention to risk management issues is important [I]. Risk management considerations include the need for collaboration and communication with any other treating clinicians as well as the need for careful and adequate documentation. Any problems with transference and countertransference should be attended to, and consultation with a colleague should be considered for unusually high-risk patients. Standard guidelines for terminating treatment should be followed in all cases. Psychoeducation about the disorder is often appropriate and helpful. Other clinical features requiring particular consideration of risk management issues are the risk of suicide, the potential for boundary violations, and the potential for angry, impulsive, or violent behavior.

II. FORMULATION AND IMPLEMENTATION OF A TREATMENT PLAN

When the psychiatrist first meets with a patient who may have borderline personality disorder, a number of important issues related to differential diagnosis, etiology, the formulation, and treatment planning need to be considered. The psychiatrist performs an initial assessment to determine the treatment setting, completes a comprehensive evaluation (including differential diagnosis), and works with the patient to mutually establish the treatment framework. The psychiatrist also attends to a number of principles of psychiatric management that form the foundation of care for patients with borderline personality disorder. The psychiatrist next considers several principles of treatment selection (e.g., type, focus, number of clinicians to involve). Finally, the psychiatrist selects specific treatment strategies for the clinical features of borderline personality disorder.

A. THE INITIAL ASSESSMENT

1. Initial assessment and determination of the treatment setting

The psychiatrist first performs an initial assessment of the patient and determines the treatment setting (e.g., inpatient or outpatient). Since patients with borderline personality disorder commonly experience suicidal ideation (and 8%–10% commit suicide), safety issues should be given priority in the initial assessment (see section II.B.1., "Responding to Crises and Safety Monitoring," for a further discussion of this issue). A thorough safety evaluation should be done before a decision can be reached about whether outpatient, inpatient, or another level of care (e.g., partial hospitalization or residential care) is needed. Presented here are some of the more common indications for particular levels of care. However, this list is not intended to be exhaustive. Since indications for level of care are difficult to empirically investigate and studies are lacking, these recommendations are derived primarily from expert clinical opinion.

Indications for partial hospitalization (or brief inpatient hospitalization if partial hospitalization is not available) include the following:

- Dangerous, impulsive behavior unable to be managed with outpatient treatment
- Nonadherence with outpatient treatment and a deteriorating clinical picture
- Complex comorbidity that requires more intensive clinical assessment of response to treatment
- Symptoms of sufficient severity to interfere with functioning, work, or family life that are unresponsive to outpatient treatment

Indications for brief inpatient hospitalization include the following:

- Imminent danger to others
- Loss of control of suicidal impulses or serious suicide attempt

- Transient psychotic episodes associated with loss of impulse control or impaired judgment
- Symptoms of sufficient severity to interfere with functioning, work, or family life that are unresponsive to outpatient treatment and partial hospitalization

Indications for extended inpatient hospitalization include the following:

- Persistent and severe suicidality, self-destructiveness, or nonadherence to outpatient treatment or partial hospitalization
- Comorbid refractory axis I disorder (e.g., eating disorder, mood disorder) that presents a potential threat to life
- Comorbid substance abuse or dependence that is severe and unresponsive to outpatient treatment or partial hospitalization
- Continued risk of assaultive behavior toward others despite brief hospitalization
- Symptoms of sufficient severity to interfere with functioning, work, or family life that are unresponsive to outpatient treatment, partial hospitalization, and brief hospitalization

2. Comprehensive evaluation

Once an initial assessment has been done and the treatment setting determined, a more comprehensive evaluation should be completed as soon as clinically feasible. Such an evaluation includes assessing the presence of comorbid disorders, degree and type of functional impairment, needs and goals, intrapsychic conflicts and defenses, developmental progress and arrests, adaptive and maladaptive coping styles, psychosocial stressors, and strengths in the face of stressors (see Part B, section V.B., "Assessment"). The psychiatrist should attempt to understand the biological, interpersonal, familial, social, and cultural factors that affect the patient (3).

Special attention should be paid to the differential diagnosis of borderline personality disorder versus axis I conditions (see Part B, sections V.A.2., "Comorbidity," and V.C., "Differential Diagnosis"). Treatment planning should address comorbid disorders from axis I (e.g., substance use disorders, depressive disorders, PTSD) and axis II as well as borderline personality disorder, with priority established according to risk or predominant symptoms. When priority is given to treating comorbid conditions (e.g., substance abuse, depression, PTSD, or an eating disorder), it may be helpful to caution patients or their families about the expected rate of response or extent of improvement. The prognosis for treatment of these axis I disorders is often poorer when borderline personality disorder is present. It is usually better to anticipate realistic problems than to encourage unrealistically high hopes.

3. Establishing the treatment framework

It is important at the outset of treatment to establish a clear and explicit treatment framework. This is sometimes called "contract setting." While this process is generally applicable to the treatment of all patients, regardless of diagnosis, such an agreement is particularly important for patients with borderline personality disorder. The clinician and the patient can then refer to this agreement later in the treatment if the patient challenges it.

Patients and clinicians should establish agreements about goals of treatment sessions (e.g., symptom reduction, personal growth, improvement in functioning) and what role each is expected to perform to achieve these goals. Patients, for example, are expected to report on such issues as conflicts, dysfunction, and impending life changes. Clinicians are expected to offer understanding, explanations for treatment interventions, undistracted attention, and respectful, compassionate attitudes, with judicious feedback to patients that can help them attain their goals. In addition, it is essential for patients and clinicians to work toward establishing agreements about 1) when, where, and with what frequency sessions will be held; 2) a plan for crises management; 3) clarification of the clinician's after-hours availability; and 4) the fee, billing, and payment schedule.

B. PRINCIPLES OF PSYCHIATRIC MANAGEMENT

Psychiatric management forms the foundation of psychiatric treatment for patients with borderline personality disorder. It consists of an array of ongoing activities and interventions that should be instituted for all patients. These include providing education about borderline personality disorder, facilitating adherence to a psychotherapeutic or psychopharmacological regimen that is satisfactory to both the patient and psychiatrist, and attempting to help the patient solve practical problems, giving advice and guidance when needed.

Specific components of psychiatric management are discussed here as well as additional important issues—such as the potential for splitting and boundary problems—that may complicate treatment and of which the clinician must be aware and manage.

1. Responding to crises and safety monitoring

Psychiatrists should assume that crises, such as interpersonal crises or self-destructive behavior, will occur. Psychiatrists may wish to establish an explicit understanding about what they expect a patient to do during crises and may want to be explicit about what the patient can expect from them. While some clinicians believe that this is of critical importance (4, 5), others believe that this approach is too inflexible and potentially adversarial. From the latter perspective, there is often a tension between the psychiatrist's role in helping patients to understand their behavior and the psychiatrist's role in ensuring patients' safety and in managing problematic behaviors. This tension may be particularly prominent when the psychiatrist is using a psychodynamic approach that relies heavily on interpretation and exploration. Regardless of the psychotherapeutic strategy, however, the psychiatrist has a fundamental responsibility to monitor this tension as part of the treatment process.

Patients with borderline personality disorder commonly experience suicidal ideation and are prone to make suicide attempts or engage in self-injurious behavior (e.g., cutting). Monitoring patients' safety is a critically important task. It is important that psychiatrists always evaluate indicators of self-injurious or suicidal ideas and reformulate the treatment plan as appropriate. Serious self-harm can occur if the potential danger is ignored or minimized. Before intervening to prevent self-endangering behaviors, the psychiatrist should first assess the potential danger, the patient's motivations, and to what extent the patient can manage his or her safety without external interventions (6). When the patient's safety is judged to be at serious risk, hospitalization may be indicated. Even in the context of appropriate treatment, some patients with borderline personality disorder will commit suicide.

2. Establishing and maintaining a therapeutic framework and alliance

Patients with borderline personality disorder have difficulty developing and sustaining trusting relationships. This issue may be a focus of treatment as well as a significant barrier to the development of the treatment alliance necessary to carry out the treatment plan. Therefore, the psychiatrist should pay particular attention to ascertaining that the patient agrees with and accepts the treatment plan; adherence or agreement cannot be assumed. Agreements should be explicit.

The first aspect of alliance building, referred to earlier as "contract setting," is establishing an agreement about respective roles and responsibilities and treatment goals. The next aspect of alliance building is to encourage patients to be actively engaged in the treatment, both in their tasks (e.g., monitoring medication effects or noting and reflecting on their feelings) and in the relationship (e.g., disclosing reactions or wishes to the clinician). This can be accomplished by focusing attention on whether the patient 1) understands and accepts what the psychiatrist says and 2) seems to feel understood and accepted by the psychiatrist. Techniques such as confrontation or interpretation may be appropriate over the long term after a "working alliance" (collaboration over a task) has been established. Psychotherapeutic approaches are often helpful in developing a working alliance for a pharmacotherapy component of the treatment plan. Reciprocally, the experience of being helped by medication that the psychiatrist prescribed can help a patient develop trust in his or her psychotherapeutic interventions.

3. Providing education about the disorder and its treatment

Psychoeducational methods often are helpful and generally are welcomed by patients and, when appropriate, their families. At an appropriate point in treatment, patients should be familiarized with the diagnosis, including its expected course, responsiveness to treatment, and, when appropriate, pathogenic factors. Many patients with borderline personality disorder profit from ongoing education about self-care (e.g., safe sex, potential legal problems, balanced diet). Formal psychoeducational approaches may include having the patient read the text of DSM-IV-TR or books on borderline personality disorder written for laypersons. Some clinicians prefer to frame psychoeducational discussions in everyday terms and use the patient's own language to negotiate a shared understanding of the major areas of difficulty without turning to a text or manual. More extensive psychoeducational intervention, consisting of workshops, lectures, or seminars, may also be helpful.

Families or others—especially those who are younger—living with individuals with borderline personality disorder will also often benefit from psychoeducation about the disorder, its course, and its treatment. It is wise to introduce information about pathogenic issues that may involve family members with sensitivity to the information's likely effects (e.g., it may evoke undesirable reactions of guilt, anger, or defensiveness). Psychoeducation for families should be distinguished from family therapy, which is sometimes a desirable part of the treatment plan and sometimes not, depending on the patient's history and status of current relationships.

4. Coordinating the treatment effort

Providing optimal treatment for patients with borderline personality disorder who may be dangerously self-destructive frequently requires a treatment team that involves several clinicians. If the team members work collaboratively, the overall treatment will usually be enhanced by being better able to help patients contain their acting out (via fight or flight) and their projections onto others. It is essential that ongoing coordination of the overall treatment plan is assured by clear role definitions, plans for management of crises, and regular communication among the clinicians.

The team members must also have a clear agreement about which clinician is assuming the primary overall responsibility for the patient's safety and treatment. This individual serves as a gatekeeper for the appropriate level of care (whether it be hospitalization, residential treatment, or day hospitalization), oversees the family involvement, makes decisions regarding which potential treatment modalities are useful or should be discontinued, helps assess the impact of medications, and monitors the patient's safety. Because of the diversity of knowledge and expertise required for this oversight function, a psychiatrist is usually optimal for this role.

5. Monitoring and reassessing the patient's clinical status and treatment plan

With all forms of treatment, it is important to monitor the treatment's effectiveness in an ongoing way. Often the course of treatment is uneven, with periodic setbacks (e.g., at times of stress). Such setbacks do not necessarily indicate that the treatment is ineffective. Nonetheless, ultimate improvement should be a reasonably expected outcome.

a) Recognizing functional regression. Patients with borderline personality disorder sometimes regress early in treatment as they begin to engage in the treatment process, getting somewhat worse before they get better. However, sustained deterioration is a problem that requires attention. Examples of such regressive phenomena include dysfunctional behavior (e.g., cessation of work, increased suicidality, onset of compulsive overeating) or immature behavior. This may occur when patients believe that they no longer need to be as responsible for taking care of themselves, thinking that their needs can and will now be met by those providing treatment.

Clinicians should be prepared to recognize this effect and then explore with patients whether their hope for such care is realistic and, if so, whether it is good for their long-term welfare. When the decline of functioning is sustained, it may mean that the focus of treatment needs to shift from exploration to other strategies (e.g., behavioral modification, vocational counseling, family education, or limit setting). Of special significance is that such declines in function are likely to occur when patients with borderline personality disorder have reductions in the intensity or amount of support they receive, such as moving to a less intensive level of care. Clinicians need to be alert to the fact that such regressions may reflect the need to add support or structure temporarily to the treatment by way of easing the transition to less intensive treatment. Regressions may also occur when patients perceive particularly sympathetic, nurturant, or protective inclinations in those who are providing their care. Under these circumstances, clinicians need to clarify that these inclinations do not signify a readiness to take on a parenting role.

b) Treating symptoms that reappear despite continued pharmacotherapy. An issue that frequently requires assessment and response by psychiatrists is the sustained return of symptoms, the previous remission of which had been attributed, at least in part, to medications (although placebo effects may also have been involved). Assessment of such symptom "breakthroughs" requires knowledge of the patient's symptom presentation before the use of medication. Has the full symptom presentation returned? Are the current symptoms sustained over time, or do they reflect transitory and reactive moods in response to an interpersonal crisis? Medications can modulate the intensity of affective, cognitive, and impulsive symptoms, but they should not be expected to extinguish feelings of anger, sadness, and pain in response to separations, rejections, or other life stressors. When situational precipitants are identified, the clinician's primary focus should be to facilitate improved coping. Frequent medication changes in pursuit of improving transient mood states are unnecessary and generally ineffective. The patient should not be given the erroneous message that emotional responses to life events are merely biologic symptoms to be regulated by medications.

c) Obtaining consultations. Clinicians with overall or primary responsibilities for patients with borderline personality disorder should have a low threshold for seeking consultation because of 1) the high frequency of countertransference reactions and medicolegal liability complications; 2) the high frequency of complicated multitreater, multimodality treatments; and 3) the particularly high level of inference, subjectivity, and life/death significance that clinical judgments involve. The principle that should guide whether a consultation is obtained is that improvement (e.g., less distress, more adaptive behaviors, greater trust) is to be expected during treatment. Thus, failure to show improvement in targeted goals by 6–12 months should raise considerations of introducing changes in the treatment. When a patient continues to do poorly after the treatment has been modified, consultation is indicated as a way of introducing and implementing treatment changes. When a consultant believes that the existing treatment cannot be improved, this offers support for continuing this treatment.

6. Special issues

a) Splitting. The phenomenon of "splitting" signifies an inability to reconcile alternative or opposing perceptions or feelings within the self or others, which is characteristic of borderline personality disorder. As a result, patients with borderline personality disorder tend to see people or situations in "black or white," "all or nothing," "good or bad" terms. In clinical settings, this phenomenon may be evident in their polarized but alternating views of others as either idealized (i.e., "all good") or devalued (i.e., "all bad"). When they perceive primary clinicians as "all bad" (usually prompted by feeling frustrated), this may precipitate flight from treatment. When splitting threatens continuation of the treatment, clinicians should be prepared to examine the transference and countertransference and consider altering treatment. This can be done by offering increased support, by seeking consultation, or by otherwise suggesting changes in the treatment. Clinicians should always arrange to communicate regularly about their patients to avoid splitting within the treatment team (i.e., one clinician or treatment is idealized while another is devalued). Integration of the clinicians helps patients integrate their internal splits.

b) Boundaries. Clinicians/therapists vary considerably in their tolerance for patient behaviors (e.g., phone calls, silences) and in their expectations of the patient (e.g., promptness, personal disclosures, homework between sessions). It is important to be explicit about these issues, thereby establishing "boundaries" around the treatment relationship and task. It is also important to be consistent with agreed-upon boundaries. Although patients may agree to such boundaries, some patients with borderline personality disorder will attempt to cross them (e.g., request between-session contacts or seek a personal, nonprofessional relationship). It remains the therapist's responsibility to monitor and sustain the treatment boundaries. Certain situations—e.g., practicing in a small community, rural area, or military setting—may complicate the task of maintaining treatment boundaries (7).

To diminish the problems associated with boundary issues, clinicians should be alert to their occurrence. Clinicians should then be proactive in exploring the meaning of the boundary crossing—whether it originated in their own behavior or that of the patient. After efforts are made to examine the meaning, whether the outcome is satisfactory or not, clinicians should restate their expectations about the treatment boundaries and their rationale. If the patient keeps testing the agreed-upon framework of therapy, clinicians should explicate its rationale. An example of this rationale is, "There are times when I may not answer your personal questions if I think it would be better for us to know why you've inquired." If a patient continues to challenge the framework despite exploration and clarification, a limit will eventually need to be set. An example of setting a limit is, "You recall that we agreed that if you feel suicidal, then you will go to an emergency room. If you cannot do this then your treatment may need to be changed."

When a boundary is crossed by the clinician/therapist, it is called a boundary "violation." The boundary can usually be restored with comments like the following: "If I were to call you every time I'm worried, your safety might come to depend too much on my intuition," or "Whenever I tell you something about my personal life, it limits our opportunity to understand more about what you imagine in the absence of knowing." When therapists find themselves making exceptions to their usual treatment boundaries, it is important to examine their motives (see section IV., "Risk Management Issues"). It often signals the need for consultation or supervision.

Any consideration of sexual boundary violations by therapists must begin with a caveat: Patients can never be blamed for ethical transgressions by their therapists. It is the therapist's responsibility to act ethically, no matter how the patient may behave. Nevertheless, specific transference-countertransference enactments are at high risk for occurring with patients with borderline personality disorder. If a patient has experienced neglect and abuse in childhood, he or she may wish for the therapist to provide the love the patient missed from parents. Therapists may have rescue fantasies that lead them to collude with the patient's wish for the therapist to offer that love. This collusion in some cases leads to physical contact and even inappropriate physical contact between therapist and patient. Clinicians should be alert to these dynamics and seek consultation or personal psychotherapy or both whenever there is a risk of a boundary violation. Sexual interactions between a therapist and a patient are always unethical. When this type of boundary violation occurs, the therapist should immediately refer the patient to another therapist and seek consultation or personal psychotherapy.

C. PRINCIPLES OF TREATMENT SELECTION

1. Type

Certain types of psychotherapy (as well as other psychosocial modalities) and certain psychotropic medications are effective for the treatment of borderline personality disorder. Although it has not been empirically established that one approach is more effective than another, clinical experience suggests that most patients with borderline personality disorder will need some form of extended psychotherapy in order to resolve interpersonal problems and attain and maintain lasting improvements in their personality and overall functioning. Pharmacotherapy often has an important adjunctive role, especially for diminution of targeted symptoms such as affective instability, impulsivity, psychotic-like symptoms, and self-destructive behavior. However, pharmacotherapy is unlikely to have substantial effects on some interpersonal problems and some of the other primary features of the disorder. Although no studies have compared a combination of psychotherapy and pharmacotherapy with either treatment alone, clinical experience indicates that many patients will benefit most from a combination of psychotherapy and pharmacotherapy.

2. Focus

Patients with borderline personality disorder frequently have comorbid axis I and other axis II conditions. The nature of certain borderline characteristics often complicates the treatment provided, even when treatment is focused on a comorbid axis I condition. For example, chronic self-destructive behaviors in response to perceived abandonment, marked impulsivity, or difficulties in establishing a therapeutic alliance have been referred to as "therapy-interfering behaviors." Treatment planning should address comorbid axis I and axis II disorders as well as borderline personality disorder, with priority established according to risk or predominant symptoms. The coexisting presence of borderline personality disorder with axis I disorders is associated with a poorer outcome of a number of axis I conditions. Treatment should usually be focused on both axis I and axis II disorders to facilitate the treatment of axis I conditions as well as address problematic, treatment-interfering personality features of borderline personality disorder itself. For patients with axis I conditions and coexisting borderline traits who do not meet full criteria for borderline personality disorder, it may be sufficient to focus treatment on the axis I conditions alone, although the therapy should be monitored and the focus changed to include the borderline traits if necessary to ensure the success of the treatment.

3. Flexibility

Features of borderline personality disorder are of a heterogeneous nature. Some patients, for example, display prominent affective instability, whereas others exhibit marked impulsivity or antisocial traits. The many possible combinations of comorbid axis I and axis II disorders further contribute to the heterogeneity of the clinical picture. Because of this heterogeneity, and because of each patient's unique history, the treatment plan needs to be flexible, adapted to the needs of the individual patient. Flexibility is also needed to respond to the changing characteristics of patients over time (e.g., at one point, the treatment focus may be on safety, whereas at another, it may be on improving relationships and functioning at work). Similarly, the psychiatrist may need to use different treatment modalities or refer the patient for adjunctive treatments (e.g., behavioral, supportive, or psychodynamic psychotherapy) at different times during the treatment.

4. Role of patient preference

Successful treatment is a collaborative process between the patient and the clinician. Patient preference is an important factor to consider when developing an individual treatment plan. The psychiatrist should explain and discuss the range of treatments available for the patient's condition, the modalities he or she recommends, and the rationale for having selected them. He or she should take time to elicit the patient's views about this provisional treatment plan and modify it to the extent feasible to take into account the patient's views and preferences. The hazard of nonadherence makes it worthwhile to spend whatever time may be required to gain the patient's assent to a viable treatment plan and his or her agreement to collaborate with the clinician(s) before any therapy is instituted.

5. Multiple- versus single-clinician treatment

Treatment can be provided by more than one clinician, each performing separate treatment tasks, or by a single clinician performing multiple tasks; both are viable approaches to treating borderline personality disorder. When there are multiple clinicians on the treatment team, they may be involved in a number of tasks, including individual psychotherapy, pharmacotherapy, group therapy, family therapy, or couples therapy or be involved as administrators on an inpatient unit, partial hospital setting, halfway house, or other living situation. Such treatment has a number of potential advantages. For example, it brings more types of expertise to the patient's treatment, and multiple clinicians may better contain the patient's self-destructive tendencies. However, because of patients' propensity for engaging in "splitting" (i.e., seeing one clinician as "good" and another as "bad") as well as the real-world difficulties of maintaining good collaboration with all other clinicians, the treatment has the potential to become fragmented. For this type of treatment to be successful, good collaboration of the entire treatment team and clarity of roles are essential (7). Regardless of whether treatment involves multiple clinicians or a single therapist, its effectiveness should be monitored over time, and it should be changed if the patient is not improving.

D. SPECIFIC TREATMENT STRATEGIES FOR THE CLINICAL FEATURES OF BORDERLINE PERSONALITY DISORDER

Although there is a long clinical tradition of treating borderline personality disorder, there are no well-designed studies comparing pharmacotherapy with psychotherapy. Nor are there any systematic investigations of the effects of combined medication and psychotherapy to either modality alone. Hence, in this section we will consider psychotherapy and pharmacotherapy separately, knowing that in clinical practice the two treatments are frequently combined. Indeed, many of the pharmacotherapy studies included patients with borderline personality disorder who were also in psychotherapy, and many patients in psychotherapy studies were also taking medication. A good deal of clinical wisdom supports the notion that carefully focused pharmacotherapy may enhance the patient's capacity to engage in psychotherapy.

1. Psychotherapy

Two psychotherapeutic approaches have been shown to have efficacy in randomized controlled trials: psychoanalytic/psychodynamic therapy and dialectical behavior therapy. We emphasize that these are psychotherapeutic *approaches* because the trials that have demonstrated efficacy (8–10) have involved sophisticated therapeutic programs rather than simply the provision of individual psychotherapy. Both approaches have three key features: 1) weekly meetings with an individual therapist, 2) one or more weekly group sessions, and 3) meetings between therapists for consultation/supervision. No results are available from direct comparisons of the two approaches to suggest which patients may respond better to which modality.

Psychoanalytic/psychodynamic therapy and dialectical behavior therapy are described in more detail in Part B of this guideline (see section VI.B., "Review of Psychotherapy and Other Psychosocial Treatments"). One characteristic of both dialectical behavior therapy and psychoanalytic/psychodynamic therapy involves the length of treatment. Although brief therapy has not been systematically tested for patients with borderline personality disorder, the studies of extended treatment suggest that substantial improvement may not occur until after approximately 1 year of psychotherapeutic intervention has been provided and that many patients require even longer treatment.

In addition, clinical experience suggests that there are a number of "common features" that help guide the psychotherapist who is treating a patient with borderline personality disorder, regardless of the specific type of therapy used. The psychotherapist must emphasize the building of a strong therapeutic alliance with the patient to withstand the frequent affective storms within the treatment (11, 12). This process of building a positive working relationship is greatly enhanced by careful attention to specific goals for the treatment that both patient and therapist view as reasonable and attainable. Consolidation of a therapeutic alliance is facilitated as well by the establishment of clear boundaries within and around the treatment. Clinicians may find it useful to keep in mind that often patients will attempt to redefine, cross, or even violate boundaries as a test to see whether the treatment situation is safe enough for them to reveal their feelings to the therapist. Regular meeting times with firm expectation of attendance and participation are important as well as an understanding of the relative contributions of patient and therapist to the treatment process (12).

Therapists need to be active, interactive, and responsive to the patient. Self-destructive and suicidal behaviors need to be actively monitored. As seen in Figure 1, some therapists create a hierarchy of priorities to be considered in the treatment. For example, practitioners of dialectical behavior therapy (5) might consider suicidal behaviors first, followed by behaviors that interfere with therapy and then behaviors that interfere with quality of life. Practitioners of psychoanalytic or psychodynamic therapy (4, 13) might construct a similar hierarchy.

Many patients with borderline personality disorder have experienced considerable childhood neglect and abuse, so an empathic validation of the reality of that mistreatment and the suffering it has caused is a valuable intervention (12, 14–17). This process of empathizing with the patient's experience is also valuable in building a stronger therapeutic alliance (11) and paving the way for interpretive comments.

While validating patients' suffering, therapists must also help them take appropriate responsibility for their actions. Many patients with borderline personality disorder who have experienced trauma in the past blame themselves. Effective therapy helps patients realize that while they were not responsible for the neglect and abuse they experienced in childhood, they *are* currently responsible for controlling and preventing self-destructive patterns in the present. Psychotherapy can become derailed if there is too much focus on past trauma instead of attention to current functioning and problems in relating to others. Most therapists believe that interventions like interpretation, confrontation, and clarification should focus more on here-and-now situations than on the distant past (18). Interpretations of the here and now as it links to events in the past is a particularly useful form of interpretation for helping patients learn about the tendency toward repetition of maladaptive behavior patterns throughout their lives. Moreover, therapists must have a clear expectation of change as they help patients understand the origins of their suffering.

Because patients with borderline personality disorder possess a broad array of strengths and weaknesses, flexibility is a crucial aspect of effective therapy. At times therapists may be able to offer interpretations of unconscious patterns that help the patient develop insight. At other times, support and empathy may be more therapeu-

FIGURE 1. Treatment Priorities of Two Psychotherapeutic Approaches for Patients With Borderline Personality Disorder[a]

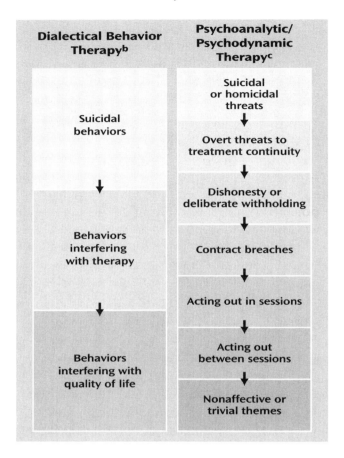

[a]Specific behaviors that practitioners of each approach may encounter in patients with borderline personality disorder are presented, with those of highest priority sitting atop the "ladder"; treatment priority lessens as one goes down the ladder.
[b]As described by Linehan et al. (5).
[c]As described by Kernberg et al. (4) and Clarkin et al. (13).

tic. Supportive strategies should not be misconstrued as simply offering a friendly relationship. Validation or affirmation of the patient's experience, strengthening of adaptive defenses, and specific advice are examples of useful supportive approaches. Interpretive or exploratory comments often work synergistically with supportive interventions. Much of the action of the therapy is focused in the therapeutic relationship, and therapists must directly address unrealistic negative and, at times, unrealistic positive perceptions that patients have about the therapist to keep these perceptions from disrupting the treatment.

Appropriate management of intense feelings in both patient and therapist is a cornerstone of good psychotherapy (15). Consulting with other therapists, enlisting the help of a supervisor, and engaging in personal psychotherapy are useful methods of increasing one's capacity to contain these powerful feelings.

Clinical experience suggests that effective therapy for patients with borderline personality disorder also involves promoting reflection rather than impulsive action.

Therapists should encourage the patient to engage in a process of self-observation to generate a greater understanding of how behaviors originate from internal motivations and affect states rather than coming from "out of the blue." Similarly, psychotherapy involves helping patients think through the consequences of their actions so that their judgment improves.

As previously noted, splitting is a major defense mechanism of patients with borderline personality disorder. The self and others are often regarded as "all good" or "all bad." This phenomenon is closely related to what Beck and Freeman (19) call "dichotomous thinking" and what Linehan (17) refers to as "all or none thinking." Psychotherapy must be geared to helping the patient begin to experience the shades of gray between the extremes and integrate the positive and negative aspects of the self and others. A major thrust of psychotherapy is to help patients recognize that their perception of others, including the therapist, is a *representation* rather than how they really are.

Because of the potential for impulsive behavior, therapists must be comfortable with setting limits on self-destructive behaviors. Similarly, at times therapists may need to convey to patients the limits of the therapist's own capacities. For example, therapists may need to lay out what they see as the necessary conditions to make therapy viable, with the understanding that the particular therapy may not be able to continue if the patient cannot adhere to minimal conditions that make psychotherapy possible.

Individual psychodynamic therapy without concomitant group therapy or other partial hospital modalities has some empirical support (20, 21). These studies, which used nonrandomized waiting list control conditions and "pre-post" comparisons, suggested that twice-weekly psychodynamic therapy for 1 year may be helpful for many patients with borderline personality disorder. In these studies, as in the randomized controlled trials, the therapists met regularly for group consultation.

There is a large clinical literature describing psychoanalytic/psychodynamic individual therapy for patients with borderline personality disorder (12, 14, 15, 18, 22–38). Most of these clinical reports document the difficult transference and countertransference aspects of the treatment, but they also provide considerable encouragement regarding the ultimate treatability of borderline personality disorder. Therapists who persevere describe substantial improvement in well-suited patients. Some of these skilled clinicians have reported success with the use of psychoanalysis four or five times weekly (22, 24, 34, 39). These cases may have involved "higher level" patients with borderline personality disorder who more likely fit into the Kernberg category of borderline personality organization (a broader theoretical rubric that describes a specific intrapsychic structural organization [27]). Some exceptional patients who do meet criteria for borderline personality disorder may be analyzable in the hands of gifted and well-trained clinicians, but most psychotherapists and psychoanalysts agree that psychoanalytic psychotherapy, at a frequency of one to three times a week face-to-face with the patient, is a more suitable treatment than psychoanalysis.

The limited literature on group therapy for patients with borderline personality disorder indicates that group treatment is not harmful and may be helpful, but it does not provide evidence of any clear advantage over individual psychotherapy. In general, group therapy is usually used in combination with individual therapy and other types of treatment, reflecting clinical wisdom that the combination is more effective than group therapy alone. Studies of combined individual dynamic therapy plus group therapy suggest that nonspecified components of combined interventions may have the greatest therapeutic power (40). Clinical experience suggests that a relatively homogeneous group of patients with borderline personality disorder is generally recommended for group therapy, although patients with dependent, schizoid, and narcissistic personality disorders or chronic depression also mix well with patients with borderline personality disorder (12). It is generally recommended that patients with antisocial personality disorder, untreated substance abuse, or psychosis not be included in groups designed for patients with borderline personality disorder.

The published literature on couples therapy with patients with borderline personality disorder consists only of reported clinical experience and case reports. This clinical literature suggests that couples therapy may be a useful and at times essential adjunctive treatment modality, since inherent in the very nature of the illness is the potential for chaotic interpersonal relationships. However, couples therapy is not recommended as the only form of treatment for patients with borderline personality disorder. Clinical experience suggests that it is relatively contraindicated when either partner is unable to listen to the other's criticisms or complaints without becoming too enraged, terrified, or despairing (41).

There is only one published study of family therapy for patients with borderline personality disorder (12), which found that a psychoeducational approach could greatly enhance communication and diminish conflict about independence. Published clinical reports differ in their recommendations about the appropriateness of family therapy and family involvement in the treatment. Whereas some clinicians recommend removing the patient's treatment from the family setting and not attempting family therapy (12), others recommend working with the patient and family together (42).

Clinical experience suggests that family work is most apt to be helpful and can be of critical importance when patients with borderline personality disorder have significant involvement with, or are financially dependent on, the family. Failure to enlist family support is a common reason for treatment dropout. The decision about whether to work with the family should depend on the degree of pathology within the family and strengths and weaknesses of the family members. Clinical experience suggests that a psychoeducational approach may lay the groundwork for the small subset of families for whom subsequent dynamic family therapy may be effective. Family therapy is not recommended as the only form of treatment for patients with borderline personality disorder.

2. Pharmacotherapy and other somatic treatments

A pharmacological approach to the treatment of borderline personality disorder is based upon evidence that some personality dimensions of patients appear to be mediated by dysregulation of neurotransmitter physiology and are responsive to medication (43). Pharmacotherapy is used to treat state symptoms during periods of acute decompensation as well as trait vulnerabilities. Although medications are widely used to treat patients who have borderline personality disorder, the Food and Drug Administration has not approved any medications specifically for the treatment of this disorder.

Pharmacotherapy may be guided by a set of basic assumptions that provide the theoretical rationale and empirical basis for choosing specific treatments. First, borderline personality disorder is a chronic disorder. Pharmacotherapy has demonstrated significant efficacy in many studies in diminishing symptom severity and optimizing functioning. However, cure is not a realistic goal—medications do not cure character. Second, borderline personality disorder is characterized by a number of dimensions; treatment is symptom-specific, directed at particular behavioral dimensions, rather than the disorder as a whole. Third, affective dysregulation and impulsive aggression are dimensions that require particular attention because they are risk factors for suicidal behavior, self-injury, and assaultiveness and are thus given high priority in selecting pharmacological agents. Fourth, pharmacotherapy targets the neurotransmitter basis of behavioral dimensions, affecting both acute symptomatic expression (e.g., anger treated with dopamine-blocking agents) and chronic vulnerability (e.g., temperamental impulsivity treated with serotonergic agents). Last, symptoms common to both axis I and II disorders may respond similarly to the same medication.

Symptoms exhibited within three behavioral dimensions seen in patients with borderline personality disorder are targeted for pharmacotherapy: affective dysregulation, impulsive-behavioral dyscontrol, and cognitive-perceptual difficulties.

a) Treatment of affective dysregulation symptoms. Affective dysregulation in patients with borderline personality disorder is manifested by symptoms such as mood lability, rejection sensitivity, inappropriate intense anger, depressive "mood crashes," and temper outbursts. As seen in Table 2, patients displaying these features should be treated initially with one of the SSRIs, since this recommendation has strong empirical support (44–49). SSRIs have a broad spectrum of therapeutic effects, are relatively safe in overdose (compared with the tricyclic antidepressants or MAOIs), and have a favorable side effect profile, which supports treatment adherence. For example, fluoxetine has been found to improve depressed mood, mood lability, rejection sensitivity, impulsive behavior, self-mutilation, hostility, and even psychotic features. Research trials of SSRIs for treatment of borderline personality disorder have ranged in duration from 6 to 14 weeks for acute treatment studies, with continuation studies lasting up to 12 months. Some patients have retained improvement with maintenance treatment of 1–3 years. Studies have been reported with fluoxetine (in doses of 20–80 mg/day), sertraline (in doses of 100–200 mg/day), and the mixed norepinephrine/serotonin reuptake blocker venlafaxine (in doses of up to 400 mg/day) (45). A reasonable trial of an SSRI for treatment of patients with borderline personality disorder is at least 12 weeks.

Empirical trials of tricyclic antidepressants have produced inconsistent results (50, 51). Patients with comorbid major depression and borderline personality disorder have shown improvement following treatment with tricyclic antidepressants. However, in one placebo-controlled study, amitriptyline had a paradoxical effect in patients with borderline personality disorder, increasing suicidal ideation, paranoid thinking, and assaultiveness (50).

Since affective dysregulation is a dimension of temperament in patients with borderline personality disorder and not an acute illness, the duration of continuation and maintenance phases of pharmacotherapy cannot presently be defined. Significant improvement in the quality of the patient's coping skills and interpersonal relationships may be required before medication can be discontinued. Clinical experience suggests caution in discontinuing a successful antidepressant trial, especially if prior medication trials have failed. In the event of a suboptimal response to an SSRI, consideration should be given to switching to a second SSRI or related antidepressant. In one study of patients with borderline personality disorder (45), one-half of the patients who failed to respond to fluoxetine subsequently responded to sertraline.

TABLE 2. Psychopharmacological Treatment Recommendations for Affective Dysregulation Symptoms in Patients With Borderline Personality Disorder

Drug Class	Specific Medications Studied	Symptoms for Which Medication Is Recommended	Strength of Evidence[a]	Issues
SSRIs and related antidepressants	Fluoxetine, sertraline, venlafaxine[b]	Depressed mood, mood lability, rejection sensitivity, anxiety, impulsivity, self-mutilation, anger/hostility, psychoticism, and poor global functioning	A	Relatively safe in overdose; favorable side effect profile; evidence obtained from acute (6–14 weeks), continuation (up to 12 months), and maintenance (1–3 years) treatment trials; second SSRI trial may still be effective if first trial fails ("salvage strategy," strength of evidence=C)
MAOIs	Phenelzine, tranylcypromine	Mood reactivity, rejection sensitivity, impulsivity, irritability, anger/hostility, atypical depression, hysteroid dysphoria	B	Second-line treatment after SSRI failure; complete elimination of initial SSRI required before MAOI treatment; adherence to required dietary restrictions problematic; effective for atypical depression only when borderline personality disorder is secondary, not primary, diagnosis
Mood stabilizers	Lithium carbonate	Mood lability, mood swings, anger, suicidality, impulsivity, poor global functioning	C	Can be used as primary or adjunctive treatment (overlaps with treatment of impulsive-behavioral domain); narrow margin of safety in overdose; blood level monitoring required; risk of hypothyroidism; to date, best studied of the mood stabilizers in treatment of personality disorders, but older literature focuses on reduction of impulsive behavior
	Carbamazepine	Suicidality, anxiety, anger, impulsivity	C	Efficacy in patients exhibiting hysteroid dysphoria; can precipitate melancholic depression; risk of bone marrow suppression; blood draws required to monitor WBC count
	Valproate	Global symptom severity, depressed mood, anger, impulsivity, rejection sensitivity, irritability, agitation, aggression, anxiety	C	Paucity of research support for this indication despite widespread use; blood draws required to monitor liver function
Benzodiazepines[c]	Alprazolam, clonazepam	Refractory anxiety, impulsivity, agitation	C	Risk of abuse, tolerance; alprazolam associated with behavioral dyscontrol
Neuroleptics[c]	Haloperidol	Behavioral dyscontrol, anger/hostility, assault, self-injury	A	Rapid onset of effect provides immediate control of behavior

[a]Ratings used by Jobson and Potter (2): A=supported by two or more randomized, placebo-controlled, double-blind trials; B=supported by at least one randomized, placebo-controlled, double-blind trial; C=supported by open-label studies, case reports, and studies that do not meet standards of randomized, placebo-controlled, double-blind trials. See text for specific supporting studies.
[b]A mixed norepinephrine/serotonin reuptake blocker.
[c]Agents primarily used as adjunctive treatment.

When affective dysregulation appears as anxiety, an SSRI may be insufficient. At this point, the use of a benzodiazepine should be considered, although there is little systematic research on the use of these medications in patients with borderline personality disorder. Use of benzodiazepines may be problematic, given the risk of abuse, tolerance, and even behavioral toxicity. Despite clinical use of benzodiazepines (52), the short-acting benzodiazepine alprazolam was associated in one study with serious behavioral dyscontrol (53). Case reports demonstrate some utility for the long half-life benzodiazepine clonazepam (54). Clinical experience suggests that this medication, if used over the longer term, is best used adjunctively with an SSRI.

In theory, buspirone may treat anxiety or impulsive aggression without the risk of abuse or tolerance. However, the absence of an immediate effect generally makes this drug less acceptable to patients with borderline personality disorder. Currently, there are no published data on the use of buspirone for the treatment of affective dysregulation symptoms in patients with borderline personality disorder.

When affective dysregulation appears as disinhibited anger that coexists with other affective symptoms, SSRIs are the treatment of first choice. Fluoxetine has been shown to be effective for anger in patients with borderline personality disorder independent of its effects on depressed mood (44). Effects of fluoxetine on anger and impulsivity may appear within days, much earlier than antidepressant effects. Clinical experience suggests that in patients with severe behavioral dyscontrol, low-dose neuroleptics can be added to the regimen for a rapid response; they may also improve affective symptoms (50). Augmentation with neuroleptics should be considered before trying an MAOI, which requires more patient cooperation and adherence.

The efficacy of MAOIs for affective dysregulation symptoms in patients with borderline personality disorder has strong empirical support (55, 56). However, they are not a first-line treatment because of concerns about adherence to required dietary restrictions and because of their more problematic side effects. The effectiveness of MAOIs is supported by randomized controlled studies in patients with a primary diagnosis of borderline personality disorder as well as syndromes (e.g., atypical depression) in which the diagnosis of borderline personality disorder is considered secondary (57). MAOI antidepressants have demonstrated efficacy for impulsivity, mood reactivity, rejection sensitivity, anger, and hostility. They may also be effective for atypical depression and "hysteroid dysphoria." If a psychiatrist wishes to use an MAOI as a second-line treatment for symptoms of affective dysregulation, care should be taken to allow an adequate washout period after discontinuing SSRIs, particularly those with a long half-life.

Mood stabilizers are another second-line (or adjunctive) treatment for affective dysregulation symptoms in patients with borderline personality disorder. Lithium carbonate, carbamazepine, and valproate have been used for treatment of mood instability in patients with an axis II disorder, but there is a surprising paucity of empirical support for their use in borderline personality disorder, although studies are currently under way. Lithium carbonate has the most research support in randomized controlled trials studying patients with personality disorders (although not specifically borderline personality disorder). However, these studies focused primarily on impulsivity and aggression rather than mood regulation (58–60). Nonetheless, lithium may be helpful for mood lability as a primary presentation in patients with a personality disorder (61). Lithium has the disadvantage of a narrow margin of safety in overdose and the risk of hypothyroidism with long-term use.

Carbamazepine has demonstrated efficacy for impulsivity, anger, suicidality, and anxiety in patients with borderline personality disorder and hysteroid dysphoria (62). However, a small, controlled study of patients with borderline personality disorder with no axis I affective disorder found no significant benefit for carbamazepine (63). Carbamazepine has been reported to precipitate melancholic depression in patients with borderline personality disorder who have a history of this disorder (64), and it has the potential to cause bone marrow suppression.

Valproate demonstrated modest efficacy for depressed mood in patients with borderline personality disorder in one small, randomized, controlled trial (65). Open-label case reports suggest that this medication may also decrease agitation, aggression, anxiety, impulsivity, rejection-sensitivity, anger, and irritability in patients with borderline personality disorder (66). Although the use of carbamazepine and valproate is widespread, psychiatrists should be aware of the lack of solid research support for their use in patients with borderline personality disorder.

Although there is a paucity of data on the efficacy of ECT for patients with borderline personality disorder, much of the available data suggest that depressed patients with a personality disorder generally have a poorer outcome with ECT than depressed patients without a personality disorder. Clinical experience suggests that while ECT may sometimes be indicated for patients with borderline personality disorder and severe axis I depression that has been resistant to pharmacotherapy, affective features of the borderline diagnosis are unlikely to respond to ECT.

b) Treatment of impulsive-behavioral dyscontrol symptoms. As seen in Table 3, SSRIs are the treatment of choice for impulsive, disinhibited behavior in patients with borderline personality disorder. Randomized controlled trials and open-label studies with fluoxetine and sertraline have shown that their effect on impulsive behavior is independent of their effect on depression and anxiety (67). The effect of SSRIs on impulsivity may appear earlier than the effect on depression, with onset of action within days in some reports. Similarly, discontinuation of an SSRI following successful treatment may result in the reemergence of impulsive aggression within days. Clinical experience suggests that the duration of treatment following improvement of impulsive aggression should be determined by the clinical state of the patient, including his or her risk of exposure to life stressors and progress in learning coping skills. When the target for treatment is a trait vulnerability, a predetermined limit on treatment duration cannot be set.

When behavioral dyscontrol poses a serious threat to the patient's safety, it may be necessary to add a low-dose neuroleptic to the SSRI. Although this combination has not been studied, randomized controlled trials of neuroleptics alone have demonstrated their efficacy for impulsivity in patients with borderline personality disorder. The effect is rapid in onset, often within hours with oral use (and more rapidly when given intramuscularly), providing immediate control of escalating impulsive-aggressive behavior.

If an SSRI is ineffective, a trial of another SSRI or related antidepressant may be considered, although there are no published studies of this approach with impulsivity as a target symptom.

Clinical experience suggests that partial efficacy of an SSRI may be enhanced by adding lithium carbonate, although this combination has not been studied in patients with borderline personality disorder. Nonetheless, studies in impulsive adults and adolescents with criminal behavior (who were not selected for having borderline personality disorder) demonstrate that lithium alone is effective for impulsive-aggressive

TABLE 3. Psychopharmacological Treatment Recommendations for Impulsive-Behavioral Dyscontrol Symptoms in Patients With Borderline Personality Disorder

Drug Class	Specific Medications Studied	Symptoms for Which Medication Is Recommended	Strength of Evidence[a]	Issues
SSRIs and related antidepressants	Fluoxetine, sertraline	Impulsive aggression, anger, irritability, self-injurious behavior, poor global functioning	A	Effects on anger and impulsive aggression may appear earlier and independently of effects on depressed mood and anxiety; no published literature on second "salvage" trials if first trial fails to reduce impulsive behavior
MAOIs	Phenelzine, tranylcypromine	Anger, irritability; impulsivity in patients with hysteroid dysphoria	A	Second-line treatment after SSRI failure; complete elimination of initial SSRI required before MAOI treatment; adherence to required dietary restrictions problematic
Mood stabilizers	Lithium carbonate	Impulsive aggression in patients with related personality disorders, impulsive behavior in patients with borderline personality disorder	A	Can be used as primary or adjunctive treatment (overlaps with treatment of affective dysregulation domain); older literature does not address borderline personality disorder; toxicity a concern in overdose; blood monitoring necessary; risk of hypothyroidism with long-term use
	Carbamazepine	Impulsivity in patients with hysteroid dysphoria	C	Risk of precipitating melancholic depression reported; blood monitoring required
	Valproate	Impulsive aggression, agitation; for adolescents with disruptive behavior disorders: tension, anxiety, chronic temper outbursts, poor global functioning	C	Paucity of research support for this indication despite widespread use; one randomized, placebo-controlled, double-blind trial is under way
Atypical neuroleptics	Clozapine	Severe self-mutilation, psychoticism	C	Risk of agranulocytosis renders clozapine treatment a last resort for this indication; blood monitoring required
Typical neuroleptics (low-dose)[b]	Haloperidol	Acute anger, hostility, assaultiveness, self-injury	A	Nonspecific effects on impulsivity as adjunctive agent; more specific effects on anger; rapid onset of effect provides immediate control of escalating impulsive symptoms

[a]Ratings used by Jobson and Potter (2): A=supported by two or more randomized, placebo-controlled, double-blind trials; B=supported by at least one randomized, placebo-controlled, double-blind trial; C=supported by open-label studies, case reports, and studies that do not meet standards of randomized, placebo-controlled, double-blind trials. See text for specific supporting studies.
[b]Agents primarily used as adjunctive treatment.

symptoms (58–60). If an SSRI is ineffective, switching to an MAOI antidepressant may be considered, although it is critical to have an adequate washout period. In a placebo-controlled crossover study of women with borderline personality disorder and hysteroid dysphoria, tranylcypromine was effective for the treatment of impulsive behavior (55). In another randomized controlled trial, phenelzine was effective for the treatment of anger and irritability (56, 68). On the basis of these findings, MAOIs are recommended for treatment of impulsivity, anger, and irritability in patients with borderline personality disorder. Combining MAOIs with valproate would also appear to be rational for selected patients, although there are no studies of these combinations.

Although the use of MAOIs in patients with borderline personality disorder is supported by randomized controlled trials, because of safety considerations many clinicians prefer to use mood stabilizers for treatment of impulsive behavior. The use of carbamazepine or valproate for impulse control in patients with borderline personality disorder appears to be widespread in clinical practice, although empirical evidence for their efficacy for impulsive aggression is limited and inconclusive. Carbamazepine has been shown to decrease behavioral impulsivity in patients with borderline personality disorder and hysteroid dysphoria. However, in a small controlled study that excluded patients with an affective disorder (63), carbamazepine proved no better than placebo for impulsivity in borderline personality disorder. Support for the use of valproate for impulsivity in borderline personality disorder is derived only from case reports, one small randomized control study, and one open-label trial in which impulsivity significantly improved (65, 66, 69, 70). Preliminary evidence suggests that the atypical neuroleptics may have some efficacy for impulsivity in patients with borderline personality disorder, especially severe self-mutilation and other impulsive behaviors arising from psychotic thinking. One open-label trial (71) and one case report (72) support the use of clozapine for this indication. The difficulties and risks involved in using clozapine (e.g., neutropenia) generally warrant its use only after other treatments have failed. The newer atypical neuroleptics have fewer risks, but there are few published data on their efficacy. Further investigation is warranted for their use as a treatment for refractory impulsive aggression in patients with borderline personality disorder.

Opioid antagonists (e.g., naltrexone) are sometimes used in an attempt to decrease self-injurious behavior in patients with borderline personality disorder. However, empirical support for this approach is very preliminary, since their efficacy has been demonstrated only in case reports and small case series.

c) Treatment of cognitive-perceptual symptoms. As seen in Table 4, low-dose neuroleptics are the treatment of choice for these symptoms. This recommendation is strongly supported by randomized, double-blind controlled studies and open-label trials involving a variety of neuroleptics in both inpatient and outpatient settings and in adult and adolescent populations (50, 51, 55, 73–78).

Low-dose neuroleptics appear to have a broad spectrum of efficacy in acute use, improving not only psychotic-like symptoms but also depressed mood, impulsivity, and anger/hostility. Treatment effects appear within days to several weeks. Patients with cognitive symptoms as a primary complaint respond best to the use of low-dose neuroleptics. Patients with borderline personality disorder with prominent affective dysregulation and labile, depressive moods, in whom cognitive-perceptual distortions are secondary mood-congruent features, may do less well with neuroleptics alone. In this case, treatments more effective for affective dysregulation should be

TABLE 4. Psychopharmacological Treatment Recommendations for Cognitive-Perceptual Symptoms in Patients With Borderline Personality Disorder

Drug Class	Specific Medications Studied	Symptoms for Which Medication Is Recommended	Strength of Evidence[a]	Issues
Typical neuroleptics (low-dose)	Haloperidol, perphenazine, thiothixene, thioridazine, flupentixol, loxapine, chlorpromazine, trifluoperazine	Ideas of reference, illusions, and paranoid ideation (and associated anger/hostility); global symptom severity, depressed mood, anxiety, impulsivity, recurrent suicidal behavior	A	Effects demonstrated in short-term studies (e.g., 5–16 weeks); poor tolerance over longer trials (e.g., 22 weeks) with increased akinesia, depression; reduction of recurrent parasuicidal behaviors reported in one long-term (6-month) study; risk of tardive dyskinesia with maintenance treatment
Atypical neuroleptics	Clozapine, olanzapine, risperidone	In theory, same as for typical neuroleptics as well as self-mutilation and severe, neuroleptic-resistant psychoticism	C	No published randomized, placebo-controlled, double-blind trials in support of this indication despite widespread use; risk of agranulocytosis renders clozapine treatment a last resort for this indication
SSRIs[b]		Irritability, anger/hostility, depressed mood, impulsive aggression	A	Especially effective if affective symptoms are present; overlaps with treatment of affective dysregulation and impulsive-behavioral dyscontrol domains
MAOIs[b]		Same as for SSRIs	A	Adherence to required dietary restrictions problematic

[a]Ratings used by Jobson and Potter (2): A=supported by two or more randomized, placebo-controlled, double-blind trials; B=supported by at least one randomized, placebo-controlled, double-blind trial; C=supported by open-label studies, case reports, and studies that do not meet standards of randomized, placebo-controlled, double-blind trials. See text for specific supporting studies.
[b]Agents primarily used as adjunctive treatment.

considered. Duration of treatment may be guided by the length of treatment trials in the literature, which are generally up to 12 weeks. Prolonged use of neuroleptic medication alone in patients with borderline personality disorder (i.e., up to 22 weeks in one study) has been associated with progressive nonadherence and dropout from treatment (68, 79). There is currently a paucity of research on the use of neuroleptic medication as long-term maintenance therapy for patients with borderline personality disorder, although many clinicians regularly use low-dose neuroleptics to help patients manage their vulnerability to disruptive anger. One longer-term study (80) found that a depot neuroleptic was effective for recurrent parasuicidal behaviors in patients with borderline personality disorder. The risk of tardive dyskinesia must be weighed carefully against perceived prophylactic benefit if maintenance strategies are considered (although this risk may be lessened by the use of atypical neuroleptics).

If response to treatment with low-dose neuroleptics is suboptimal after 4 to 6 weeks, the dose should be increased into a range suitable for treating axis I disorders and continued for a second trial period of 4 to 6 weeks. A suboptimal response at this point should prompt rereview of the etiology of the cognitive-perceptual symptoms. If the symptom presentation is truly part of a nonaffective presentation, atypical neuroleptics may be considered. Although there are no published randomized controlled trials of atypical neuroleptics in patients with borderline personality disorder, open-label trials and case studies support the use of clozapine for patients with severe, refractory psychotic symptoms "of an atypical nature" or for severe self-mutilation (71, 72, 81). However, clozapine is best used in patients with refractory borderline personality disorder, given the risk of agranulocytosis. Studies are currently under way with olanzapine and risperidone (82, 83). The generally favorable side effect profiles of risperidone and olanzapine, compared with those of traditional neuroleptics, indicate that these medications warrant careful empirical trials. As yet, there are no published data on the efficacy of quetiapine for borderline personality disorder.

Neuroleptics are often effective for anger and hostility regardless of whether these symptoms occur in the context of cognitive-perceptual symptoms or other types of symptoms. It is important to note that both MAOI and SSRI antidepressants have also been shown in randomized controlled trials to be effective for irritability and anger in some patients with borderline personality disorder with cognitive-perceptual symptoms.

III. SPECIAL FEATURES
INFLUENCING TREATMENT

A. COMORBIDITY

Other disorders may be comorbid with borderline personality disorder, such as mood disorders, substance-related disorders, eating disorders (notably, bulimia), PTSD, other anxiety disorders, dissociative identity disorder, and attention deficit hyperactivity disorder (ADHD) (see section V.A.2., "Comorbidity," and refer to relevant APA Practice Guidelines [84–88]). These disorders can complicate the clinical picture and need to be addressed in treatment. Depression, often with atypical features, is particularly common in patients with borderline personality disorder (89, 90). Depressive features may meet criteria for major depressive disorder or dysthymic disorder, or they may be a manifestation of the borderline personality disorder itself. Although this distinction can be difficult to make, depressive features that appear particularly characteristic of borderline personality disorder are emptiness, self-condemnation, abandonment fears, hopelessness, self-destructiveness, and repeated suicidal gestures (91, 92). Depressive features that appear to be due to borderline personality disorder may respond to treatment approaches described in this practice guideline. Depressive features that meet criteria for major depression (especially if prominent neurovegetative symptoms are present) should be treated by using standard treatment approaches for major depression (see the APA *Practice Guideline for the Treatment of Patients With Major Depressive Disorder* [84]) in combination with treatment targeted at the borderline personality disorder. Available evidence suggests that SSRIs and MAOIs are more effective than tricyclic antidepressants for depressive features in patients with borderline personality disorder (although safety issues must be particularly carefully considered when using MAOIs).

B. PROBLEMATIC SUBSTANCE USE

Substance use disorders are common in patients with borderline personality disorder. The presence of substance use has major implications for treatment, since patients with borderline personality disorder who abuse substances generally have a poor outcome and are at greatly higher risk for suicide and for death or injury resulting from accidents. Persons with borderline personality disorder often abuse substances in an impulsive fashion that contributes to lowering the threshold for other self-destructive behavior such as body mutilation, sexual promiscuity, or provocative behavior that incites assault (including homicidal assault).

Patients with borderline personality disorder who abuse substances are seldom candid and forthcoming about the nature and extent of their abuse, especially in the early phases of therapy. For this reason, therapists should inquire specifically about substance abuse at the beginning of treatment and educate patients about the risks involved.

Vigorous treatment of any substance use disorder is essential in working with patients with borderline personality disorder (87). Depending on the severity of the alcohol abuse, if outpatient treatment is ineffective, inpatient treatment may be needed for detoxification and participation in various alcohol-treatment interventions. Participation in Alcoholics Anonymous is often helpful on both an inpatient and an outpatient basis. Clinical experience suggests that the use of disulfiram may occasionally be helpful as adjunctive treatment for patients with borderline personality disorder who use alcohol, but it must be used with caution because of the risk of impulsivity or nonadherence. Other medications effective for the treatment of alcohol abuse or dependence (e.g., naltrexone) may also be considered. Twelve-step programs are also available for persons abusing narcotics or cocaine. Opioid antagonists (e.g., naltrexone) are effective in treating opiate overdoses and are occasionally used in an attempt to decrease opiate abuse. However, they require diligent patient adherence, and there is little empirical support for the effectiveness of this approach for addiction.

Drug counseling may be a useful component of treatment. However, except perhaps for mild marijuana use, psychotherapy alone is generally ineffective for treating substance use disorders.

To the extent that various substances may be abused in order to mask depression, anxiety, and other related states, clinical experience suggests that prescribed medications—antidepressants (especially SSRIs) or nonhabituating anxiolytics such as buspirone—may help to alleviate the underlying symptoms, thus lessening the temptation to resort to the use of alcohol or drugs.

C. VIOLENT BEHAVIOR AND ANTISOCIAL TRAITS

Some patients with borderline personality disorder engage in violent behaviors. Violence may take such forms as hurling objects at family members—or at therapists—during moments of intense anger or frustration. Others may commit physical assaults. Some patients with borderline personality disorder are physically abusive toward their children. Patients with antisocial traits may engage in robbery, burglary, and car theft. Acts of this sort are often associated with an arrest record.

Therapeutic strategies optimal for dealing with antisocial features vary, depending on the severity of these features, and range from minor interventions to broader and more complex strategies suitable for a clinical picture in which antisociality is a major factor.

When antisocial features are mild (e.g., occasional shoplifting at times of severe stress), clinical experience suggests that individual cognitive therapy may be successful (e.g., encouraging the patient to weigh the risks versus the benefits—and the short-term versus the long-term consequences—of various antisocial choices the patient had been contemplating as well as identifying alternative coping strategies). This becomes in effect a psychoeducative approach in which the patient is helped to understand the advantages, in the long term, of socially appropriate alternatives (93).

When more severe antisocial features are present, residential treatment may be indicated. This may take the form of the "therapeutic community" as described by Losel (94) and by Dolan et al. (95). Various forms of group therapy are a mainstay of this approach. When episodic outbursts of violent behavior are present, the use of mood-stabilizing medications or an SSRI may be indicated (59, 96).

When antisocial features are even more severe and become dominant, and when the threat of violence is imminent, psychotherapy of any type may prove ineffective. In this situation hospitalization (involuntary, if necessary) may be required to help the patient regain control and, in cases in which a specific threat has been communicated by the patient, to reduce the risk to the potential victim(s).

Clinicians should be aware that some patients with borderline personality disorder with antisocial comorbidity may not be good candidates for therapy. This is especially true when the clinical picture is dominated by psychopathic traits (as described by Hare [97]) of the intensely narcissistic type: grandiosity, conning, lack of remorse, lying, and manipulativeness. Similarly, when underlying motives of jealousy or of revenge are of extreme intensity, therapy may prove ineffective (93).

D. CHRONIC SELF-DESTRUCTIVE BEHAVIOR

A primary feature of borderline personality disorder is impulsive self-destructive behavior, including reckless driving and spending, shoplifting, bingeing and purging, substance abuse, risky sexual behavior, self-mutilation, and suicide attempts. This behavior is thought to reflect the difficulties patients with borderline personality disorder have with modulation and containment of intense emotions or impulses. Some clinicians who are expert in the treatment of borderline personality disorder (4, 17) suggest that the psychotherapist should approach each session with a hierarchy of priorities in mind (as exhibited in Figure 1). In other words, suicidal and self-destructive behaviors would be addressed as the highest priorities, with an effort to evaluate the patient's risk for these behaviors and help the patient find ways to maintain safety. Alternatives to self-mutilation, for example, can be considered (12, 17), and insights might be offered about the meaning of self-defeating behavior. SSRIs might also be prescribed for the self-mutilating patient.

Most experts agree that some type of limit-setting is necessary at times in the treatment of patients with borderline personality disorder. Because patients engage in so many self-destructive and self-defeating behaviors, clinicians may find themselves spending a great deal of the therapy setting limits on the patient's behaviors. The risk in these situations is that therapists may become entrenched in a countertransference posture of policing the patient's behavior to the point that treatment goals are lost and the therapeutic alliance is compromised. Waldinger (18) has suggested that limit-setting should be targeted at a subgroup of behaviors, namely, those that are destructive to the patient, the therapist, or the therapy. Limit-setting is not necessarily an ultimatum involving a threat to discontinue the treatment. Therapists can indicate to the patient that certain conditions are necessary to make treatment viable.

It is also useful for psychiatrists to help the patient think through the consequences of chronic self-destructive behaviors. In this way the behavior may gradually shift from being ego syntonic to ego dystonic (i.e., the behavior becomes more distressing to the patient as he or she becomes more reflective about the adverse consequences). The patient and therapist can then form a stronger therapeutic alliance around strategies to control the behavior.

If self-destructive behaviors are relentless and out of control, and especially if patients are not willing to work on controlling such behaviors, patients may need referral to a more intensive level of care before they are able to resume outpatient treatment. Consultation may also be useful.

E. CHILDHOOD TRAUMA AND PTSD

Childhood trauma is a common although not universal feature of borderline personality disorder (98–104). Recognizing trauma-related aspects of the patient's affective instability, damaged self-image, relationship problems, fears of abandonment, self-injurious behavior, and impulsiveness is important and can facilitate psychotherapy in a variety of ways.

1. Threats to the therapeutic alliance

Recognizing a trauma history, if present, can help the therapist and patient understand current distortions in the patient's view of self and others as an understandable residual of prior life experiences that would produce mistrust. Anger, impulsiveness, and self-defeating behavior in relationships take on different meanings when understood as, in part, displaced responses to abusive early life experiences. Discounting a trauma history has the potential to undermine the therapeutic alliance and the progress of treatment. It can also hamper patients' ability to integrate and come to terms with the trauma. Not integrating traumatic material into the treatment can lead patients to experience the therapy as a form of collusion with the abuser.

2. Issues with transference

Many traumatized patients expect others, including their therapists, to be malevolent, for example, inflicting harm in the guise of providing help, analogous to a parent or other caretaker exploiting and abusing a child. This core transference mistrust may become an ongoing issue to be worked on during psychotherapy.

3. Determining appropriate treatment focus

Decisions about whether and when to focus on trauma, if present, during treatment should be based on the patient's agitation, stability, fragility, evidence of psychotic symptoms, and potential for self-harm or disruption of current vocational, family, or other roles. It is generally thought that working through the residue of trauma is best done at a later phase of treatment, after solidifying the therapeutic alliance, achieving stabilization of symptoms, and establishing an understanding of the patient's history and psychological structures (8).

4. Working through traumatic memories

In the later phase of treatment, one component of effective psychotherapy for patients with a trauma history involves exposure to, managing affect related to, and cognitively restructuring memories of the traumatic experience. This involves grief work (105), acknowledging, bearing, and putting into perspective the residue of traumatic experiences (106). This process helps to reduce the unbidden, intrusive, and alien nature of traumatic memories and differentiates affect associated with the trauma from that elicited by current relationships.

5. Importance of group support and therapy

For patients with borderline personality disorder who have experienced trauma, group work can be particularly helpful in providing support and understanding from other trauma survivors as well as a milieu in which they can gain understanding about their self-defeating behaviors and interpersonal relationship patterns. Some patients with borderline personality disorder can be less defensive receiving feedback from peers, and at certain points in therapy this may be the only place they feel understood and safe.

6. Risk of reenactment or revictimization

The vulnerability of traumatized patients to revictimization, or their deliberate incurring of risk and reenactment of early trauma, has implications for patient safety and management of the transference. The therapist should address the possibility of current or future harm to the patient.

7. Treating PTSD-like symptoms

Even when full criteria for comorbid PTSD are not present, patients with borderline personality disorder may experience PTSD-like symptoms. For example, symptoms such as intrusion, avoidance, and hyperarousal may emerge during psychotherapy. Awareness of the trauma-related nature of these symptoms can facilitate both psychotherapeutic and pharmacological efforts in symptom relief.

8. Reassignment of blame

Victims of trauma, especially early in life, typically blame themselves inappropriately for traumatic events over which they had no control (107). This may happen because the trauma was experienced during a developmental period when the child was unable to appreciate independent causation and therefore assumed he or she was responsible. Many adults blame themselves so that they avoid reexperiencing the helplessness associated with trauma. It is important in therapy to listen to a patient's guilt and sense of responsibility for past trauma and, when appropriate, to clarify the patient's lack of responsibility for past trauma as well as the importance of taking responsibility for present life circumstances.

9. Use of eye movement therapy

Eye movement desensitization and reprocessing (108) has been presented as a treatment for trauma symptoms. It involves having patients discuss a traumatic memory and then move their eyes back and forth rapidly as though they were in rapid eye movement sleep. The specific effect of the eye movements has not been established, and the treatment may mainly involve exposure to and working through trauma-related cognition and affect (109, 110). This therapy is currently under investigation. There is currently no evidence of specific efficacy for this treatment in patients with borderline personality disorder.

10. Accuracy of distant memories

Ignoring or discounting a trauma history can undermine the therapeutic alliance by aligning the therapist with individuals in the patient's past who either inflicted harm or ignored it. On the other hand, memories of remote traumatic experiences may contain inaccuracies. Dissociative symptoms may complicate retrieval of traumatic memories in patients with borderline personality disorder (111, 112). The affect may be correct even when the details about events are wrong (113). Furthermore, confrontation of family members regarding possible abusive activity is likely to produce substantial emotional response and family disruption. Thus, the approach to traumatic origins of symptoms should be open-ended, sensitive to both the effects of possible trauma and the fallibility of memory.

F. DISSOCIATIVE FEATURES

There is considerable comorbidity between borderline personality disorder and various dissociative symptoms and disorders (100, 114–117). Transient dissociative symptoms, including depersonalization, derealization, and loss of reality testing, are not uncommon and may contribute to the psychotic-like symptoms that patients with borderline personality disorder may experience. The percentage of patients with borderline personality disorder who also have dissociative identity disorder is unknown, but it is estimated that one-third of patients with dissociative identity disorder also have borderline personality disorder (118). Dissociative symptoms and dissociative identity disorder may appear as or exacerbate other borderline personality disorder characteristics, including identity disturbance, impulsivity, recurrent suicidal behavior, and affective instability. Thus, to manage these symptoms, identification of and attention to comorbid dissociative identity disorder or prominent dissociative symptoms is mandated. This includes the following:

- Exploring the extent of the dissociative symptoms
- Exploring current issues that may lead to dissociative episodes
- Clarifying the nature of dissociative symptoms and distinguishing them from malingering or deception on the one hand and psychotic symptoms on the other
- Teaching the patient how to access and learn to control dissociation, including the possible use of hypnosis in patients with full dissociative disorder
- Working through any possible posttraumatic symptoms associated with the dissociative symptoms
- Facilitating integration of dissociated identities or personality states and integrating amnesic episodes by explaining to patients that the problem is one of fragmentation of personality structure elements; practicing with the patient more fluid transitions among various identities and personality states
- Working through transference issues related to trauma and feelings about controlling dissociative symptoms
- Consolidating and stabilizing gains by providing positive reinforcement for integrated function and consistent response to dissociative components of the personality structure
- Supporting the patient in case of relapse

When borderline personality disorder and dissociative identity disorder coexist, clinical reports suggest that hypnosis may be useful for identifying and controlling dissociative symptoms (119–121). These symptoms can be reconceptualized as uncontrolled hypnotic-like states that can be elicited and modulated with hypnosis, both as a technique in therapy and as a self-hypnotic exercise to be practiced by patients under the therapist's supervision.

A crucial element in working through issues of transference/countertransference and limit-setting is the extent to which the patient is consciously aware and in control of mental states in which impulsive behavior or strong emotion are experienced. Treatment of comorbid dissociative symptoms can help to delineate the areas of available control and expand the patient's repertoire of adaptive symptom-control skills.

G. PSYCHOSOCIAL STRESSORS

In borderline personality disorder, stress may be a contributing factor in the disorder's etiology and a precipitant of symptomatic exacerbation (122). Physical or sexual abuse is not uncommon during childhood for these patients; histories of other forms of trauma, such as verbal abuse or neglect (123) and early parental separation or loss (124), are frequently elicited as well. In addition, most patients with borderline personality disorder are acutely sensitive to psychosocial stressors, particularly interpersonal stressors. Self-esteem is often fragile, and patients seek to shore up their sense of self by "borrowing" a stable, established identity from another (usually idealized) person. Relationships are intense, and everyday distractions or inattention can be interpreted as abandonment, resulting in panic-like anxiety, impulsive self-destructive acts, excessive anger, paranoia, or dissociative episodes. These sensitivities are important in therapy, since regardless of the type of treatment, once a therapeutic relationship has developed, it will take on this overdetermined, intense quality. The psychiatrist should be alert, nimble, flexible, and on the lookout for ways in which the limits of the therapeutic relationship may stimulate anxiety-driven reactions in the patient—reactions that may be confrontational, depressive, or invisible until revealed by self-destructive or impulsive acting out.

H. GENDER

Borderline personality disorder is diagnosed predominantly in women, with an estimated gender ratio of 3:1. The disorder may be missed in men, who may instead receive diagnoses of antisocial or narcissistic personality disorder. Men should be as carefully assessed for borderline personality disorder as women. The diagnostic assessment of the patient should include a detailed inquiry regarding reproductive life history, including sexual practices and birth control.

Most treatment studies of borderline personality disorder primarily involve women. There has been little systematic investigation of gender differences in treatment response.

The treatment of pregnant and nursing women raises specific concerns regarding the use of psychotropic medications. The potential risks, which are highest during the first trimester of pregnancy, have been reviewed elsewhere (125). When treating women with borderline personality disorder who are pregnant or nursing, the risks of treatment with medication must be carefully weighed against the potential risks and benefits of alternative treatment (e.g., psychotherapy alone) as well as the risk to the women if the borderline personality disorder and comorbid conditions are not treated (125, 126). These potential risks and benefits should be discussed with the patient.

Because anticonvulsants are associated with a potential risk of birth defects, and the risk of birth defects from other psychotropic medications is unknown, psychiatrists should encourage careful contraceptive practices for all female patients of childbearing age who are receiving pharmacological treatment. Since carbamazepine can increase the metabolism of birth control pills, the dosage of oral contraceptives may need to be adjusted accordingly. Whenever possible, planned pregnancy should be pursued in consultation with the psychiatrist so that options, including maintenance of pharmacological treatment or discontinuation of these agents, can be thoughtfully pursued. For patients who become pregnant while on a maintenance regimen of psychiatric medications, a consultation for further consideration of the relative risks of continuing or discontinuing medications should also be considered (127, 128).

Gender issues, including psychotropic medication use during pregnancy, that are associated with certain comorbid conditions are discussed in other APA Practice Guidelines (84–86).

I. CULTURAL FACTORS

Borderline personality disorder has been reported in many cultures around the world (129). The cultural context of a patient's presentation should be considered. Cultural factors may hamper the accurate assessment of borderline personality disorder. An appreciation by the clinician of cultural variables is critical in making an accurate diagnosis. Clinicians should be especially careful to avoid cultural bias when applying the diagnostic criteria and evaluating sexual behavior, expressions of emotion, or impulsiveness, which may have different norms in different cultures.

Ethnic groups may differ in their response to psychotropic medications. Although inconclusive, some studies have suggested that Asian patients may require lower doses of haloperidol and have higher serum levels of haloperidol after oral administration than Caucasian patients (130). Psychiatrists should be aware of this possibility when administering neuroleptic medication to Asian patients. Some studies also suggest that ethnic groups may differ in their response to antidepressant medications (131, 132).

J. AGE

Because the personality of adolescents is still developing, the diagnosis of borderline personality disorder should be made with care in this age group. Borderline personality disorder may be present in the elderly, although later in life a majority of individuals with this disorder attain greater stability in functioning. Virtually no treatment studies have been done in adolescents or elderly persons with borderline personality disorder. Although treatments effective in adults would be expected to be efficacious in these age groups, research that demonstrates this efficacy is needed, especially in adolescents. It should be kept in mind that elderly patients are particularly prone to certain medication side effects (e.g., orthostatic hypotension and anticholinergic effects) and therefore may tolerate certain medications less well than younger adults.

IV. RISK MANAGEMENT ISSUES

A. GENERAL CONSIDERATIONS

When treating patients with any mental disorder, attention to risk management issues is important and often enhances patient care. Attention to these issues is particularly important when treating patients with borderline personality disorder, given the potential for self-injury, violent behavior, and suicide, as well as impulsivity, splitting, problems with the therapeutic alliance, and transference and countertransference problems (e.g., the mobilization of intense feelings in the clinician). The following are general risk management considerations for patients with borderline personality disorder:

- Good collaboration and communication with other clinicians who are also treating the patient is necessary.
- Attention should be paid to careful and adequate documentation, including assessment of risk, communication with other clinicians, the decision-making process, and the rationale for the treatment used.
- Attention should be paid to any transference and countertransference problems that have the potential to cloud good clinical judgment. The clinician should be especially aware of the potential for splitting to occur and should resist taking on the role of the "all good" or rescuing clinician. In this regard, close collaboration and communication with other team members is important. Keep in mind that different perspectives of different clinicians can be valid, since the patient may act differently with different clinicians.
- Consultation with a colleague should be considered and may be useful for unusually high-risk patients (e.g., when suicide risk is very high), when the patient is not improving, or when it is unclear what the best treatment approach might be. It is important to document the consultation (i.e., that the consultation has occurred, what the recommendations were, whether the recommendations were followed or not, and, if the clinician made a different treatment decision, why the recommendations were not followed).
- Termination of treatment with a patient with borderline personality disorder must be managed with care. Standard guidelines for terminating psychiatric treatment should be followed, even if it is the patient's decision to terminate treatment (133). Careful attention must be paid to timing, transfer, and discussion with the patient. If the treatment termination process is unusually difficult or complex, obtaining a consultation should be considered.
- Psychoeducation about the disorder is often appropriate and helpful from both a clinical and risk management perspective. When appropriate, family members should be included, with attention to confidentiality issues. Psychoeducation should include discussion of the risks inherent in the disorder and the uncertainties of the treatment outcome.

B. SUICIDE

Suicidal threats, gestures, and attempts are very common among patients with borderline personality disorder, and 8%–10% commit suicide. Managing suicide risk therefore poses important clinical and medicolegal challenges for clinicians. However, it can be difficult to address suicide risk in these patients for a number of reasons. First, suicidality can be acute, chronic, or both, and responses to these types of suicidality differ in some ways. Second, given the tendency of patients with borderline personality disorder to be chronically suicidal and to engage in self-destructive behaviors, it can be difficult to discern when a patient is at imminent risk of making a serious suicide attempt. Third, even with careful attention to suicide risk, it is often difficult to predict serious self-harm or suicide, since this behavior can occur impulsively and without warning. Fourth, given the potential for difficulties in forming a good therapeutic alliance, it may be difficult to work collaboratively with the patient to protect him or her from serious self-harm or suicide. Last, even with good treatment, some patients will commit suicide. The following are risk management considerations for suicidal behavior in patients with borderline personality disorder:

- Monitor patients carefully for suicide risk and document this assessment; be aware that feelings of rejection, fears of abandonment, or a change in the treatment may precipitate suicidal ideation or attempts.
- Take suicide threats seriously and address them with the patient. Taking action (e.g., hospitalization) in an attempt to protect the patient from serious self-harm is indicated for acute suicide risk.
- Chronic suicidality without acute risk needs to be addressed in therapy (e.g., focusing on the interpersonal context of the suicidal feelings and addressing the need for the patient to take responsibility for his or her actions). If a patient with chronic suicidality becomes acutely suicidal, the clinician should take action in an attempt to prevent suicide.
- Actively treat comorbid axis I disorders, with particular attention to those that may contribute to or increase the risk of suicide (e.g., major depression, bipolar disorder, alcohol or drug abuse/dependence).
- If acute suicidality is present and not responding to the therapeutic approaches being used, consultation with a colleague should be considered.
- Consider involving the family (if otherwise clinically appropriate and with adequate attention to confidentiality issues) when patients are chronically suicidal. For acute suicidality, involve the family or a significant other if their involvement will potentially protect the patient from harm.
- A promise to keep oneself safe (e.g., a "suicide contract") should not be used as a substitute for a careful and thorough clinical evaluation of the patient's suicidality with accompanying documentation. However, some experienced clinicians carefully attend to and intentionally utilize the negotiation of the therapeutic alliance, including discussion of the patient's responsibility to keep himself or herself safe, as a way to monitor and minimize the risk of suicide.

C. ANGER, IMPULSIVITY, AND VIOLENCE

Anger and impulsivity are hallmarks of borderline personality disorder and can be directed at others, including the clinician. This is particularly likely to occur when there is a disruption in the patient's relationships or when he or she feels abandoned (e.g., there is a change in clinicians) or when the patient feels betrayed, unjustly accused, or seriously misunderstood and blamed by the clinician or a significant other. Even with close monitoring and attention to these issues in the treatment, it is difficult to predict their occurrence. Another complicating factor is that the patient's anger or behavior may produce anger in the therapist, which has the potential to adversely affect clinical judgment. The following are risk management considerations for anger, impulsivity, and violence in patients with borderline personality disorder:

- Monitor the patient carefully for impulsive or violent behavior, which is difficult to predict and can occur even with appropriate treatment.
- Address abandonment/rejection issues, anger, and impulsivity in the treatment.
- Arrange for adequate coverage when away; carefully communicate this to the patient and document coverage.
- If the patient makes threats toward others (including the clinician) or exhibits threatening behavior, the clinician may need to take action to protect self or others.

D. BOUNDARY VIOLATIONS

With patients with borderline personality disorder there is a risk of boundary crossings and violations. The following are risk management considerations for boundary issues with patients with borderline personality disorder:

- Monitor carefully and explore countertransference feelings toward the patient.
- Be alert to deviations from the usual way of practicing, which may be signs of countertransference problems—e.g., appointments at unusual hours, longer-than-usual appointments, doing special favors for the patient.
- Always avoid boundary violations, such as the development of a personal friendship outside of the professional situation or a sexual relationship with the patient.
- Get a consultation if there are striking deviations from the usual manner of practice.

PART B:
BACKGROUND INFORMATION AND REVIEW OF AVAILABLE EVIDENCE

V. DISEASE DEFINITION, EPIDEMIOLOGY, AND NATURAL HISTORY

A. DEFINITION AND CORE CLINICAL FEATURES

The essential feature of borderline personality disorder is a pervasive pattern of instability of interpersonal relationships, affects, and self-image, as well as marked impulsivity that begins by early adulthood and appears in a variety of contexts. These characteristics are severe and persistent enough to result in clinically significant impairment in social, occupational, or other important areas of functioning. Common and important features of borderline personality disorder are a severely impaired capacity for attachment and predictably maladaptive behavior in response to separation. Individuals with this disorder are very sensitive to abandonment and make frantic efforts to avoid real or perceived abandonment. They often experience intense abandonment fears and anger in reaction to even realistic time-limited separation. Efforts to avoid abandonment may include inappropriate rage, unfair accusations, and impulsive behaviors such as self-mutilation or suicidal behaviors, which often elicit a guilty or fearful protective response from others.

The relationships of individuals with borderline personality disorder tend to be unstable, intense, and stormy. Their views of others may suddenly and dramatically shift, alternating between extremes of idealization and devaluation, or seeing others as beneficent and nurturing and then as cruel, punitive, and rejecting. These shifts are particularly likely to occur in response to disillusionment with a significant other or when a sustaining relationship is threatened or lost.

The disorder is usually characterized by identity disturbance, which consists of markedly and persistently unstable self-image or sense of self. Self-image (goals, values, type of friends, vocational goals) may suddenly and dramatically shift. Individuals with this disorder usually feel bad or evil, but they may also feel that they do not exist at all, especially when feeling unsupported and alone.

Many individuals with borderline personality disorder are impulsive in one or more potentially self-damaging areas, such as spending money irresponsibly, gambling, engaging in unsafe sexual behavior, abusing drugs or alcohol, driving recklessly, or binge eating. Self-mutilation (e.g., cutting or burning) and recurrent suicidal behaviors, gestures, or threats are common. These self-destructive acts are often precipitated by potential separation from others, perceived or actual rejection or abandonment, or the expectation from others that they assume more responsibility.

Affective instability is another common feature of the disorder. This consists of marked mood reactivity (e.g., intense episodic dysphoria, irritability, or anxiety that usually lasts for a few hours and only rarely for more than a few days). The usual dysphoric mood of these individuals is often punctuated by anger, panic, or despair and is only infrequently relieved by periods of well-being. These episodes may be triggered by the individual's extreme reactivity to interpersonal stressors. Individuals with this disorder also typically have chronic feelings of emptiness. Many experience inappropriate, intense anger or have difficulty controlling their anger. For example, they may lose their temper, feel constant anger, have verbal outbursts, or engage in physical fights. This anger may be triggered by their perception that an important person is neglectful, withholding, uncaring, or abandoning. Expressions of anger may be followed by feelings of being evil or by feelings of shame and guilt. During periods of extreme stress (e.g., perceived or actual abandonment), these individuals may experience transient paranoid ideation or severe dissociative symptoms (e.g., depersonalization).

It is not necessary for an individual to have all of the above features for borderline personality disorder to be diagnosed. As indicated in Table 1, the diagnosis is given if at least five of the nine diagnostic criteria are present.

1. Associated features

Transient psychotic-like symptoms (e.g., hearing their name called) may occur at times of stress. These episodes usually last for minutes or hours and are generally of insufficient duration or severity to warrant an additional diagnosis. Another common associated feature is a tendency for these individuals to undermine themselves when a goal is about to be reached (e.g., severely regressing after a discussion of how well therapy is going). Individuals with this disorder may feel more secure with transitional objects (e.g., a pet or inanimate object) than with interpersonal relationships. Despite their significant relationship problems, they may deny that they are responsible for such problems and may instead blame others for their difficulties.

Physical and sexual abuse, neglect, hostile conflict, and early parental loss or separation are more common in the childhood histories of those with borderline personality disorder than in those without the disorder.

2. Comorbidity

Axis I disorders and other axis II disorders are often comorbid with borderline personality disorder. Among the most commonly comorbid axis I disorders are mood disorders, substance-related disorders, eating disorders (notably bulimia), PTSD, panic disorder, and ADHD. Such axis I comorbidity can complicate and worsen the course of borderline personality disorder. Commonly co-occurring axis II disorders are antisocial, avoidant, histrionic, narcissistic, and schizotypal personality disorders.

3. Complications

Borderline personality disorder is characterized by notable distress and functional impairment. A majority of patients attempt suicide. Completed suicide occurs in 8%–10% of individuals with this disorder, a rate that is approximately 50 times higher than in the general population. Risk of suicide appears to be highest when patients are in their 20s as well as in the presence of co-occurring mood disorders or substance-related disorders (87). Physical handicaps may result from self-inflicted injury or failed suicide attempts. These individuals often have notable difficulty with occupational, academic, or role functioning. Their functioning may deteriorate in unstructured work or school situations, and recurrent job loss and interrupted education are common. Difficulties in relationships, as well as divorce, are also common.

The social cost for patients with borderline personality disorder and their families is substantial. Longitudinal studies of patients with borderline personality disorder indicate that even though these patients may gradually attain functional roles 10–15 years after admission to psychiatric facilities, still only about one-half will have stable, full-time employment or stable marriages (40, 134). Recent data indicate that patients with borderline personality disorder show greater lifetime utilization of most major categories of medication and of most types of psychotherapy than do patients with schizotypal, avoidant, or obsessive-compulsive personality disorder or patients with major depressive disorder (135).

B. ASSESSMENT

A skilled clinical interview is the mainstay of diagnosing borderline personality disorder. This approach should be complemented by knowledge of the DSM criteria and a longitudinal view of the clinical picture. The additional use of assessment instruments can be useful, especially when the diagnosis is unclear. Use of such instruments must be accompanied by clinical judgment.

Certain assessment issues relevant to all personality disorders should be considered when diagnosing borderline personality disorder. For the diagnosis to be made, the personality traits must cause subjective distress or significant impairment in functioning. The traits must also deviate markedly from the culturally expected and accepted range, or norm, and this deviation must be manifested in more than one of the following areas: cognition, affectivity, control over impulses, and ways of relating to others. Therefore, multiple domains of experience and behavior (i.e., cognition, affect, intrapsychic experience, and interpersonal interaction) must be assessed to determine whether borderline traits are distressing or impairing. The clinician should also ascertain that the personality traits are of early onset, pervasive, and enduring; they should not be transient or present in only one situation or in response to only one specific trigger. It is important that borderline personality disorder be assessed as carefully in men as in women.

The ego-syntonicity of the personality traits may complicate the assessment process; the use of multiple sources of information (e.g., medical records and informants who know the patient well) can be particularly helpful in establishing the diagnosis if the patient's self-awareness is limited. Given the high comorbidity of axis I disorders with borderline personality disorder, it is important to do a full axis I evaluation. An attempt should be made to distinguish axis I states (e.g., mood disorder) from borderline personality disorder, which can be a complex process. Useful approaches are to obtain a description of the patient's personality traits and coping styles when prominent axis I symptoms are absent and to use information provided by people who have known the patient without an axis I disorder. If axis I disorders are present, both the axis I disorders and borderline personality disorder should be diagnosed.

Because the personality of children and adolescents is still developing, borderline personality disorder should be diagnosed with care in this age group. Often, the presence of the disorder does not become clear until late adolescence or adulthood.

When assessing a patient with borderline personality disorder, the clinician should carefully look for the presence of risk-taking and impulsive behaviors, mood disturbance and reactivity, risk of suicide, risk of violence to persons or property, substance abuse, the patient's ability to care for himself/herself or others (e.g., children), financial resources, psychosocial stressors, and psychosocial supports (e.g., family and friends).

C. DIFFERENTIAL DIAGNOSIS

Borderline personality disorder often co-occurs with mood disorders, and when criteria for both are met, both should be diagnosed. However, some features of borderline personality disorder may overlap with those of mood disorders, complicating the differential diagnostic assessment. For example, the affective instability and impulsivity of borderline personality disorder may mimic features of bipolar disorder, especially bipolar II disorder. However, in borderline personality disorder, the mood swings are often triggered by interpersonal stressors (e.g., rejection), and a particular mood is usually less sustained than in bipolar disorder. Depressive features may meet criteria for major depressive disorder or may be features of the borderline personality disorder itself. Depressive features that appear particularly characteristic of borderline personality disorder are emptiness, self-condemnation, abandonment fears, self-destructiveness, and hopelessness (91, 92). It can be particularly difficult to differentiate dysthymic disorder from borderline personality disorder, given that chronic dysphoria is so common in individuals with borderline personality disorder. However, the presence of the aforementioned affective features (e.g., mood swings triggered by interpersonal stressors) should prompt consideration of the diagnosis of borderline personality disorder. In addition, the other features of borderline personality disorder (e.g., identity disturbance, chronic self-destructive behaviors, frantic efforts to avoid abandonment) are generally not characteristic of axis I mood disorders. In other cases, what appear to be features of borderline personality disorder may constitute symptoms of an axis I disorder (e.g., bipolar disorder). A more in-depth consideration of the differential diagnosis or treatment of the presumed axis I condition may help clarify such questions.

PTSD is a common comorbid condition in patients with borderline personality disorder, and, when present, should be diagnosed. However, a history of trauma is often characteristic of patients with borderline personality disorder and does not necessarily warrant an additional diagnosis of PTSD. PTSD should be diagnosed only when full criteria for the disorder are met. PTSD is characterized by rapid-onset symptoms that occur, usually in adulthood, in reaction to exposure to a recognizable and extreme stressor; in contrast, borderline personality disorder consists of the early-onset, enduring personality traits described elsewhere in this guideline.

Although borderline personality disorder may be comorbid with dissociative identity disorder, the latter (unlike borderline personality disorder) is characterized by the presence of two or more distinct identities or personality states that alternate, manifesting different patterns of behavior.

D. EPIDEMIOLOGY

Borderline personality disorder is the most common personality disorder in clinical settings. It is present in 10% of individuals seen in outpatient mental health clinics,

15%–20% of psychiatric inpatients, and 30%–60% of clinical populations with a personality disorder. It occurs in an estimated 2% of the general population (1, 136).

Borderline personality disorder is diagnosed predominantly in women, with an estimated gender ratio of 3:1. The disorder is present in cultures around the world. It is approximately five times more common among first-degree biological relatives of those with the disorder than in the general population. There is also a greater familial risk for substance-related disorders, antisocial personality disorder, and mood disorders.

E. NATURAL HISTORY AND COURSE

Long-term follow-up studies of treated patients with borderline personality disorder indicate that the course is variable. Early adulthood is often characterized by chronic instability, with episodes of serious affective and impulsive dyscontrol and high levels of use of health and mental health resources. Later in life, a majority of individuals attain greater stability in social and occupational functioning.

In the largest follow-up study to date (137), about one-third of patients with borderline personality disorder had recovered by the follow-up evaluation, having solidified their identity during the intervening years and having replaced their tendency toward self-damaging acts, inordinate anger, and stormy relationships with more mature and more modulated behavior patterns. Longitudinal studies of hospitalized patients with borderline personality disorder indicate that even though they may gradually attain functional roles 10–15 years after admission to psychiatric facilities, only about one-half of the women and one-quarter of the men will have attained enduring success in intimacy (as indicated by marriage or long-term sexual partnership) (137). One-half to three-quarters will have by that time achieved stable full-time employment. These studies concentrated on patients with borderline personality disorder from middle-class or upper-middle-class families. Patients with borderline personality disorder from backgrounds of poverty have substantially lower success rates in the spheres of intimacy and work. Despite these somewhat favorable outcomes, the suicide rate among patients with borderline personality disorder is high—approximately 9%. The risk of suicide appears highest in the young-adult years.

VI. REVIEW AND SYNTHESIS OF AVAILABLE EVIDENCE

A. ISSUES IN INTERPRETING THE LITERATURE

The following issues should be considered when interpreting the literature presented in this guideline on the efficacy of treatments for borderline personality disorder. Virtually all of the studies involved adults with borderline personality disorder. While the results may be applicable to adolescents, there is a paucity of research that has examined the efficiency of these treatments for this age group. Although some of these treatments have been evaluated through randomized, placebo-controlled trials—the gold standard for determining treatment efficacy— information for other treatments is available only from case reports, case series, or retrospective studies, which limits the conclusions that can be drawn about treatment efficacy.

Another consideration is that efficacy studies (e.g., placebo-controlled trials) have notable strengths but also some limitations. Although such studies are necessary to establish that a particular treatment is effective, there may be limits to how generalizable the study findings are. For example, inclusion and exclusion criteria result in particular types of patients being involved in a study. When reviewing the data presented in this guideline, clinicians should consider how similar their patient is to the population included in a particular study. This is particularly important because of the heterogeneous nature of borderline personality disorder symptoms. Some studies, for example, select patients with marked impulsivity, whereas others include patients with prominent affective features. In addition, many studies have been relatively short term; longer-term treatment outcome studies are needed.

Another issue to consider is that some studies are done in specialized research settings with more expertise and training in the treatment modality than is generally available in the community. In addition, the amount of treatment provided in a study may be greater than is actually available in the community.

When evaluating studies of psychosocial treatments that consist of multiple elements, such as psychodynamic psychotherapy, it may be difficult to know which elements are responsible for the treatment outcome. Another factor to consider is that patients in certain studies of psychosocial treatment were also taking prescription medication, and no steps were taken to control for these effects. Conversely, patients in some studies of medication efficacy also received psychotherapy, and no steps were taken to control for these effects. Therefore, the literature on the efficacy of any one particular treatment is often confounded by the presence of other simultaneous treatments. It can be difficult, then, to isolate the impact of a single modality in most treatment efficacy studies involving patients with borderline personality disorder.

In clinical practice, a combination of treatment approaches is often used and appropriate. Few data are available on the complex treatment regimens often required by the realities of clinical practice (e.g., the use of multiple medications simultaneously). Many clinically important and complex treatment questions have not been (and are unlikely to ever be) addressed in research studies. For such questions, clinical consensus is the best available guide.

B. REVIEW OF PSYCHOTHERAPY AND OTHER PSYCHOSOCIAL TREATMENTS

1. Psychodynamic psychotherapy

Psychodynamic psychotherapy has been defined as a therapy that involves careful attention to the therapist-patient interaction with, when indicated, thoughtfully timed interpretation of transference and resistance embedded in a sophisticated appreciation of the therapist's contribution to the two-person field. Psychodynamic psychotherapy draws from three major theoretical perspectives: ego psychology, object relations, and self psychology. Most therapeutic approaches to patients with borderline personality disorder do not adhere strictly to only one of these theoretical frameworks. The approach of Stevenson and Meares (20, 138), for example, encompasses the self-psychological ideas of Kohut and the object relations ideas of Winnicott, whereas the technique of Kernberg et al. (4, 13, 28) is based on an amalgamation of ego psychology and object relations theory.

a) Definition and goals. Psychodynamic psychotherapy is usually conceptualized as operating on an exploratory-supportive (also called expressive-supportive) continuum of interventions (Figure 2). At the more exploratory end of the continuum, the goals of psychodynamic psychotherapy with patients with borderline personality disorder are to make unconscious patterns more consciously available, to increase affect tolerance, to build a capacity to delay impulsive action, to provide insight into relationship problems, and to develop reflective functioning so that there is greater appreciation of internal motivation in self and others. From the standpoint of object relations theory, one major goal is to integrate split-off aspects of self and object representations so that the patient's perspective is more balanced (e.g., seeing others as simultaneously having both positive and negative qualities). From a self-psychological perspective, a major goal is to strengthen the self so that there is less fragmentation and a greater sense of cohesion or wholeness in the patient's self-experience. On the supportive end of the continuum, the goals involve strengthening of defenses, the shoring up of self-esteem, the validation of feelings, the internalization of the therapeutic relationship, and creation of a greater capacity to cope with disturbing feelings.

Of these interventions, only interpretation is unique to the psychodynamic approach. The more exploratory interventions (interpretation, confrontation, and clarification) may be focused on either transference or extratransference issues.

FIGURE 2. The Exploratory-Supportive Intervention Continuum of Psychodynamic Psychotherapy[a]

Interpretation	Confrontation	Clarification	Encouragement to Elaborate	Empathic Validation	Advice and Praise	Affirmation
Linking a patient's feeling, thought, behavior, or symptom to its unconscious meaning or origin	Addressing issues the patient does not want to accept or wishes to avoid	Reformulating what the patient says into a more coherent view of what is meant	Requesting more information from the patient	Demonstrating empathy with the patient's internal state	Prescribing and reinforcing certain activities of benefit to the patient	Supporting the patient's comments or behaviors

Exploratory   **Supportive**

[a]Adapted from Gabbard (139).

i) Interpretation.   Among the most exploratory forms of treatment, interpretation is regarded as the therapist's ultimate therapeutic tool. In its simplest form, interpretation involves making something conscious that was previously unconscious. An interpretation is an explanatory statement that links a feeling, thought, behavior, or symptom to its unconscious meaning or origin. For example, a therapist might make the following observation to a patient with borderline personality disorder: "I wonder if your tendency to undermine yourself when things are going better is a way to assure that your treatment with me will continue."

ii) Confrontation.   This exploratory intervention addresses something the patient does not want to accept or identifies the patient's avoidance or minimization. A confrontation may be geared to clarifying how the patient's behavior affects others or reflects a denied or suppressed feeling. An example might be, "I think talking exclusively about your medication problems may be a way of avoiding any discussion with me about your painful feelings that make you feel suicidal."

iii) Clarification.   This intervention involves a reformulation or pulling together of the patient's verbalizations to convey a more coherent view of what is being communicated. A therapist might say, "It sounds like what you're saying is that in every relationship you have, no one seems to be adequately attuned to your needs."

iv) Encouragement to elaborate.   Closer to the center of the continuum are interventions that are characteristic of both supportive and exploratory therapies. Encouragement to elaborate may be broadly defined as a request for information about a topic brought up by the patient. Simple comments like, "Tell me more about that," or, "What do you mean when you say you feel 'empty'?" are examples of this intervention.

v) Empathic validation.   This intervention is a demonstration of the therapist's empathic attunement with the patient's internal state. This approach draws from self psychology, which emphasizes the value of empathy in strengthening the self. A typically validating comment is, "I can understand why you feel depressed about that," or, "It hurts when you're treated that way."

vi) Advice and praise.   This category includes two interventions that are linked by the fact that they both prescribe and reinforce certain activities. Advice involves direct suggestions to the patient regarding how to behave, while praise reinforces certain patient behaviors by expressing overt approval of them. An example of advice would be, "I don't think you should see that man again because you get beaten up every time you're with him." An example of praise would be, "I think you used excellent judgment in breaking off your relationship with that man."

vii) Affirmation.   This simple intervention involves succinct comments in support of the patient's comments or behaviors such as, "Yes, I see what you mean," or, "What a good idea."

Some patients with borderline personality disorder receive a highly exploratory or interpretive therapy that is focused on the transference relationship. This approach is sometimes called transference-focused psychotherapy (4, 140). Patients who lack good abstraction capacity and psychological mindedness may require a therapy that is primarily supportive, even though it is psychodynamically informed by a careful analysis of the patient's ego capacities, defenses, and weaknesses. Most psychotherapies involve both exploratory and supportive elements and include some, although not exclusive, focus on the transference. Hence, psychodynamic psychotherapy is often conceptualized as exploratory-supportive or expressive-supportive psychotherapy (16, 139, 141).

b) Efficacy.   While there is a great deal of clinical literature on psychodynamic psychotherapy with patients who have borderline personality disorder, there are relatively few methodologically rigorous efficacy studies. One randomized controlled trial assessed the efficacy of psychoanalytically informed partial hospitalization treatment, of which dynamic therapy was the primary modality (9). In this study, 44 patients were randomly assigned to either the partial hospitalization program or general psychiatric care. Treatment in the partial hospitalization program consisted of weekly individual psychoanalytic psychotherapy, three-times-a-week group psychoanalytic psychotherapy, weekly expressive therapy informed by psychodrama, weekly community meetings, monthly meetings with a case administrator, and monthly medication review by a resident. The control group received general psychiatric care consisting of regular psychiatric review with a senior psychiatrist twice a month, inpatient admission as appropriate, outpatient and community follow-up, and no formal psychotherapy. The average length of stay in the partial hospitalization program was 1.5 years. Relative to the control group, the completers of the partial hospitalization program showed significant improvement: self-mutilation decreased, the proportion of patients who attempted suicide decreased from 95% before treatment to 5% after treatment, and patients improved in terms of state and trait anxiety, depression, global symptoms, social adjustment, and interpersonal problems. In the last 6 months of the study, the number of inpatient episodes and duration of inpatient length of stay dramatically increased for the control subjects, whereas these utilization variables remained stable for subjects in the partial hospitalization group.

One can conclude from this study that patients with borderline personality disorder treated with this program for 18 months showed significant improvement in terms of both symptoms and functioning. Reduction of symptoms and suicidal acts occurred after the first 6 months of treatment, but the differences in frequency and duration of inpatient treatment emerged only during the last 6 months of treatment. In addition, depressive symptoms were significantly reduced. Although the principal treatment received by subjects in the partial hospitalization group was psychoanalytic individual and group therapy, one cannot definitively attribute this group's better outcome to the type of therapy received, since the overall community support and social network within which these therapies took place may have exerted significant effects. Pharmacotherapy received was similar in the two treatment groups, but subjects in the partial hospitalization program had a greater amount of psychotherapy than did the control subjects. In a subsequent report (10), patients who had received partial hospitalization treatment not only maintained their substantial gains at an 18-month follow-up evaluation but also showed statistically significant continued improvement on most measures, whereas the control group showed only limited change during the same period.

A study from Australia of twice-weekly psychodynamic therapy (20) prospectively compared the year before 12 months of psychodynamic therapy was given with the year after the therapy was received for a group of poorly functioning outpatients with borderline personality disorder. Among the 30 completers, there were significant reductions in violent behavior, use of illegal drugs, number of medical visits, self-harm, time away from work, severity of global symptoms, number of DSM-III symptoms of borderline personality disorder, number of hospital admissions, and time spent as an inpatient. Although this study did not include a control group, there were dramatic improvements in patients that support the value of the year-long treatment intervention.

In another study (21), this same group of 30 patients who received psychodynamic therapy was compared with 30 control subjects drawn from an outpatient waiting list who then received treatment as usual, consisting of supportive therapy, cognitive therapy, and crisis intervention. The control subjects were assessed at baseline and at varying intervals, with an average follow-up duration of 17.1 months. In this nonrandomized controlled study, the group receiving psychodynamic therapy had a significantly better outcome than the control subjects (i.e., fewer subjects in the treatment versus the control group still met DSM-III criteria for borderline personality disorder), even though the group that received psychodynamic therapy was more severely ill at baseline. This study suggests that psychodynamic therapy is efficacious, but the investigation has a number of limitations, including the lack of randomization, different follow-up durations for different subjects, nonblind assessment of outcome, and lack of detail about the amount of treatment received by the control subjects. Without more data on the amount of treatment received, it is unclear whether the better outcome of the subjects who received dynamic therapy was due to the type of therapy or the greater amount of treatment received.

c) Cost-effectiveness.   The investigators of the Australian study also did a preliminary cost-benefit analysis (138) in which they compared the direct cost of treatment for the 12 months preceding psychodynamic therapy with the direct cost of treatment for the 12 months following this therapy. In Australian dollars, the cost of the treatment for all patients decreased from $684,346 to $41,424. Including psychotherapy in the cost of treatment, there was a total savings per patient of $8,431 per year. This cost-effectiveness was accounted for almost entirely by a decrease in the number of hospital days. Without a control group, however, one cannot definitively conclude that the cost savings were the result of the psychotherapy.

d) Length and frequency of treatment.   Most clinical reports of psychodynamic psychotherapy involving patients with borderline personality disorder refer to the treatment duration as "extended" or "long term." However, there are only limited data about how much therapy is adequate or optimal. In the aforementioned randomized controlled trial of psychoanalytically focused partial hospitalization treatment (9), the effect of psychotherapy on reducing hospitalization was not significant until after the patients had been in therapy for more than 12 months. There are no studies demonstrating that brief therapy or psychotherapy less than twice a week is helpful for patients with borderline personality disorder. Howard and colleagues (142), to study the psychotherapeutic dose-effect relationship, conducted a meta-analysis comprising 2,431 subjects from 15 patient groups spanning 30 years. One study they examined in detail involved a group of 151 patients evaluated by self-report and by chart review; 28 of these patients had a borderline personality disorder diagnosis. Whereas 50% of patients with anxiety or depression improved in eight to 13 sessions, the same degree of improvement occurred after 13–26 sessions for "borderline psychotic" patients according to self-ratings (the same degree of improvement occurred after

26–52 sessions according to chart ratings by researchers [143]). Seventy-five percent of patients with borderline personality disorder had improved by 1 year (52 sessions) and 87%–95% by 2 years (104 sessions). While this study confirms the conventional wisdom that more therapy is needed for patients with borderline personality disorder than for patients with an axis I disorder, it is unclear whether raters were blind to diagnosis. It appears that a standardized diagnostic assessment and standard threshold for improvement were not used, there are no data on treatment dropouts, and little information is provided about the type of therapy or the therapists except that they were predominantly psychodynamically oriented. What can be concluded is that in a naturalistic setting, outpatients who are clinically diagnosed as "borderline psychotic" will likely need more extended therapy than will depressed or anxious patients.

e) Adverse effects. While no adverse effects were reported in the aforementioned studies, psychodynamic psychotherapy has the potential to disorganize some patients if the focus is too exploratory or if there is too much emphasis on transference without an adequately strong alliance. Intensive dynamic psychotherapy may also activate strong dependency wishes in the patient as transference wishes and feelings develop in the context of the treatment. It is the exploration of such dependency that is often essential to help the patient to achieve independence. This dependence may elicit countertransference problems in the therapist, which can lead to inappropriate or ineffective treatment. The most serious examples of this include unnecessary increases in the frequency or duration of treatment or transgression of professional boundaries.

f) Implementation issues.

  i) Difficulties with adherence. Most studies report a high dropout rate from dynamic psychotherapy among patients with borderline personality disorder. However, this is true for almost all approaches to the treatment of these patients, and it has not been demonstrated to be any higher for dynamic therapy. It does, however, emphasize the paramount importance of adequate attention to the therapeutic alliance as well as to transference and countertransference issues.

  ii) Need for therapist flexibility. Early in the treatment, and periodically in the later stages, a therapist who is also functioning as primary clinician may need to take a major role in management issues, including limit-setting, attending to suicidality, addressing pharmacotherapy, and helping to arrange hospitalization. A stance in which the therapist only explores the patient's internal experience and does not become involved in management of life issues may lead to adverse outcomes for some patients.

  iii) Importance of judicious transference interpretation. Excessive transference interpretation or confrontation early in treatment may increase the risk that the patient will drop out of therapy. One process study of psychoanalytic therapy with patients with borderline personality disorder (11) found that for some patients, transference interpretation is a "high-risk, high-gain" phenomenon in that it may improve the therapeutic alliance but also may cause substantial deterioration in that alliance. Therapists must use transference interpretation judiciously on the basis of their sense of the state of the alliance and the patient's capacity to hear and reflect on observations about the therapeutic relationship. A series of empathic and supportive comments often paves the way for an effective transference interpretation. Other patients may be able to use transference interpretation effectively without this much preparatory work.

iv) Role of therapist training and competency. Psychodynamic therapy for patients with borderline personality disorder is uncommonly demanding. Consultation from an experienced colleague is highly recommended for all therapists during the course of the therapy. In some situations, personal psychotherapy can help the clinician develop skills to manage the intense transference/countertransference interactions that are characteristic of these treatments.

2. Cognitive behavior therapy

a) Definition and goals. Although cognitive behavior therapy has been widely used and described in the clinical literature, it has more often been used to treat axis I conditions (e.g., anxiety or depressive disorders) than personality disorders. Cognitive behavior therapy assumes that maladaptive and distorted beliefs and cognitive processes underlie symptoms and dysfunctional affect or behavior and that these beliefs are behaviorally reinforced. It generally involves attention to a set of dysfunctional automatic thoughts or deeply ingrained belief systems (often referred to as schemas), along with learning and practicing new, nonmaladaptive behaviors. Utilization of cognitive behavior methods in the treatment of the personality disorders has been described (19), but because persistent dysfunctional belief systems in patients with personality disorders are usually "structuralized" (i.e., built into the patient's usual cognitive organization), substantial time and effort are required to produce lasting change. Modifications of standard approaches (e.g., schema-focused cognitive therapy, complex cognitive therapy, or dialectical behavior therapy) are often recommended in treating certain features typical of the personality disorders. However, other than dialectical behavior therapy (17, 144–147), these modifications have not been studied.

b) Efficacy. Most published reports of cognitive behavior treatment for patients with borderline personality disorder are uncontrolled clinical or single case studies. Recently, however, several controlled studies have been done, particularly of a form of cognitive behavior therapy called dialectical behavior therapy. Dialectical behavior therapy consists of approximately 1 year of manual-guided therapy (involving 1 hour of weekly individual therapy for 1 year and 2.5 hours of group skills training per week for either 6 or 12 months) along with a requirement for all therapists in a study or program to meet weekly as a group. Linehan and colleagues (8) reported a randomized controlled trial of dialectical behavior therapy involving patients with borderline personality disorder whose symptoms included "parasuicidal" behavior (defined as any intentional acute self-injurious behavior with or without suicide intent). Control subjects in this study received "treatment as usual" (defined as "alternative therapy referrals, usually by the original referral source, from which they could choose"). Of the 44 study completers, 22 received dialectical behavior therapy, and 22 received treatment as usual; patients were assessed at 4, 8, and 12 months. At pretreatment, 13 of the control subjects had been receiving individual psychotherapy, and nine had not. Patients who received dialectical behavior therapy had less parasuicidal behavior, reduced medical risk due to parasuicidal acts, fewer hospital admissions, fewer psychiatric hospital days, and a greater capacity to stay with the same therapist than did the control subjects. Both groups improved with respect to depression, suicidal ideation, hopelessness, or reasons for living; there were no group differences on these variables. Because there were substantial dropout rates overall (30%) and the number of study completers in each group was small, it is unclear how generalizable these results are. Nonetheless, this study is a promising first report of a manualized regimen of cognitive behavior treatment for a specific type of patient with borderline personality disorder.

A second cohort of patients was subsequently studied; the same study design was used (148). In this report, there were 26 intent-to-treat patients (13 received dialectical behavior therapy, 13 received treatment as usual). One patient who received dialectical behavior therapy committed suicide late in the study, and three patients receiving dialectical behavior therapy and one patient receiving treatment as usual dropped out. Nine of the 13 control patients were already receiving individual psychotherapy at the beginning of the study or entered such treatment during the study. Patients who received dialectical behavior therapy had greater reduction in trait anger and greater improvement in Global Assessment Scale scores.

One year after termination of their previously described study (8), the Linehan group reevaluated their patient group (5). After 1 year, the greater reduction in parasuicide rates and in severity of suicide attempts seen in the dialectical behavior therapy group relative to the control subjects did not persist, although there were significantly fewer psychiatric hospital days for the dialectical behavior therapy group during the follow-up year. These findings suggest that although dialectical behavior therapy produces a greater reduction in parasuicidal behavior than treatment as usual, the durability of this advantage is unclear.

In a subsequent report, Linehan and colleagues (149) compared dialectical behavior therapy with treatment as usual in patients with borderline personality disorder with drug dependence. Only 18 of the 28 intent-to-treat patients completed the study (seven who received dialectical behavior therapy, 11 given treatment as usual). Patients receiving dialectical behavior therapy had more drug- and alcohol-abstinent days after 4, 8, and 16 months. All patients had reduced parasuicidal behavior as well as state and trait anger; there was no difference between the groups. This study, too, involved small numbers of patients and had substantial dropout rates, but it represents an important attempt to evaluate the impact of dialectical behavior therapy with severely ill patients with borderline personality disorder and comorbid substance abuse.

In all of these studies, it is difficult to ascertain whether the improvement reported for patients receiving dialectical behavior therapy derived from specific ingredients of dialectical behavior therapy or whether nonspecific factors such as either the greater time spent with the patients or therapist bias contributed to the results. In a small study in which skills training alone was compared with a no-skills training control condition, no difference was found between the groups (unpublished 1993 study of MM Linehan and HL Heard). The researchers concluded that the specific features of individual dialectical behavior therapy are necessary for patients to show greater improvement than control groups. Linehan and Heard (150) reported that more time with therapists does not account for improved outcome. Nonetheless, other special features of dialectical behavior therapy, such as the requirement for all therapists to meet weekly as a group, could contribute to the results.

Springer et al. (151) used an inpatient group therapy version of dialectical behavior therapy for patients with personality disorders, 13 of whom had borderline personality disorder. The patients with borderline personality disorder exhibited improvement in depression, hopelessness, and suicidal ideation, but the improvement was not greater than it was for a control group. In this study, compared with control subjects, patients receiving the dialectical behavior therapy treatment showed a paradoxical increase in parasuicidal acting out during the brief hospitalization (average length of stay was 12.6 days).

Barley and colleagues (152) compared dialectical behavior therapy received by patients with borderline personality disorder on a specialized personality disorder inpatient unit with treatment as usual on a similar-sized inpatient unit. They found that the use of dialectical behavior therapy was associated with reduced parasuicidal behavior. It is unclear whether improvement was due to dialectical behavior therapy per se or to other elements of the specialized unit.

Perris (153) reported preliminary findings from a small uncontrolled, naturalistic follow-up study of 13 patients with borderline personality disorder who received cognitive behavior therapy similar to dialectical behavior therapy. Twelve patients were evaluated at a 2-year follow-up point, and all patients maintained the normalization of functioning that had been evident at the end of the study treatment.

Other controlled studies reported in the literature of cognitive behavior approaches are difficult to interpret because of small patient group sizes or because the studies focused on mixed types of personality disorders without specifying borderline cohorts (154–156).

In summary, there are a number of studies in the literature suggesting that cognitive behavior therapy approaches may be effective for patients with borderline personality disorder. Most of these studies involved dialectical behavior therapy and were carried out by Linehan and her group. Replication studies by other groups in other centers are needed to confirm the validity and generalizability of these findings.

c) Cost-effectiveness.   Published data are not available on the cost-effectiveness of cognitive behavior approaches for treatment of borderline personality disorder, although Linehan and colleagues (8) reported that patients receiving dialectical behavior therapy had fewer psychiatric inpatient days and psychiatric hospital admissions than did control subjects.

d) Length and frequency of treatment.   Short-term cognitive therapy involving 16–20 sessions has been described as a generic treatment approach; however, the patient characteristics thought to be necessary for a successful treatment outcome are not typical of patients with personality disorders (147). Instead, longer forms of treatment, such as "schema-focused cognitive therapy" (147), "complex cognitive therapy" (144), or dialectical behavior therapy (17), are usually recommended.

The standard length of dialectical behavior therapy is approximately 1 year for the most commonly administered phase of the treatment. It involves 1 hour of individual therapy per week, more than 2 hours of group skills training per week (for either 6 or 12 months), and 1 hour of group process for the therapists per week. Other versions of dialectical behavior therapy, such as that administered in a brief inpatient setting (151), may be useful but are not necessarily more effective than other forms of inpatient treatment.

e) Adverse effects.   Although there are no reports of adverse effects of cognitive behavior therapy, including dialectical behavior therapy, as administered on an outpatient basis, one inpatient study (151) reported a paradoxical increase in parasuicidal acting out in the dialectical behavior therapy group compared with the control group—a finding thought perhaps to be due to the contagion effect within a closed, intensive milieu.

f) Implementation issues. Many components of cognitive behavior therapy are similar to elements of psychodynamic psychotherapy, although they may have different labels. For example, as Linehan (17) pointed out, focusing on "therapy-interfering behavior" is similar to the psychodynamic emphasis on transference behaviors. Similarly, the notion of validation resembles that of empathy. Beck and Freeman (19) noted that cognitive therapists and psychoanalysts have the common goal of identifying and modifying "core" personality disorder problems. However, psychodynamic therapists view these core problems as having important unconscious roots that are not available to the patient, whereas cognitive therapists view them as largely in the realm of awareness. It is not clear how successfully psychiatrists who have not been trained in cognitive behavior therapy can implement manual-based cognitive behavior approaches.

Although dialectical behavior therapy has been well described in the literature for many years, it is not clear how difficult it is to teach to new therapists in settings other than that where it was developed. Variable results in other settings could be due to a number of factors, such as less enthusiasm for the method among therapists, differences in therapist training in dialectical behavior therapy, and different patient populations. Although the Linehan group has developed training programs for therapists, certain characteristics recommended in dialectical behavior therapy (e.g., "a matter-of-fact, somewhat irreverent, and at times outrageous attitude about current and previous parasuicidal and other dysfunctional behaviors" [17]) may be more effective when carried out by therapists who are comfortable with this particular style.

3. Group therapy

a) Goals. The goals of group therapy are consistent with those of individual psychotherapy and include stabilization of the patient, management of impulsiveness and other symptoms, and examination and management of transference and countertransference reactions. Groups provide special opportunities for provision of additional social support, interpersonal learning, and diffusion of the intensity of transference issues through interaction with other group members and the therapists. In addition, the presence of other patients provides opportunities for patient-based limit setting and for altruistic interactions in which patients can consolidate their gains in the process of helping others.

b) Efficacy. Some uncontrolled studies suggest that group treatment (157), including process-focused groups in a therapeutic community setting (158), may be helpful for patients with borderline personality disorder. However, these studies had no true control condition, and the efficacy of the group treatment is unclear, given the complexity of the treatment received. Another small chart review study of an "incest group" for patients with borderline personality disorder (159) suggested shorter subsequent inpatient stays and fewer outpatient visits for treated patients than for control subjects. A randomized trial (160) involving patients with borderline personality disorder showed equivalent results with group versus individual dynamically oriented psychotherapy, but the small sample size and high dropout rate make the results inconclusive. Wilberg et al. (161) did a naturalistic follow-up study of two cohorts of patients with borderline personality disorder. This quasi-experimental, nonrandomized study showed that patients with borderline personality disorder discharged from a day program with continuing outpatient group therapy (N=12) did better than those who did not have group therapy (N=31). They had better global health and lower global severity index symptoms, lower Health-Sickness Rating Scale scores, lower SCL-90 scores, lower rehospitalization rates, fewer suicide attempts, and less substance abuse. There were, however, important differences between the two comparison groups that could account for outcome differences.

Perhaps the most interesting aspect of group therapy is the use of groups to consolidate and maintain improvement from the inpatient stay. Linehan and colleagues (8) combined individual and group therapy, making the specific effect of the group component unclear. They reported that, contrary to expectations, the addition of group skills training to individual dialectical behavior therapy did not improve clinical outcome. For those patients with borderline personality disorder who have experienced shame or have become isolated as a result of trauma, including those with comorbid PTSD, group therapy with others who have experienced trauma can be helpful. Such groups provide a milieu in which their current emotional reactions and self-defeating behaviors can be seen and understood. Groups may also provide a context in which patients may initiate healthy risk-taking in relationships. Group treatment has also been included in studies of psychodynamic psychotherapy; although the overall treatment program was effective, the effectiveness of the group therapy component is unknown (9, 162). Clinical wisdom indicates for many patients combined group and individual psychotherapy is more effective than either treatment alone.

c) Cost-effectiveness. Group psychotherapy is substantially less expensive than individual therapy because of the favorable therapist-patient ratio. Marziali and Monroe-Blum (163) calculated that group psychotherapy for borderline personality disorder costs about one-sixth as much as individual psychotherapy, assuming that the fee for individual therapy is only slightly higher than that for group therapy. However, this potential saving is tempered by the fact that most treatment regimens for borderline personality disorder combine group interventions with individual therapy.

d) Length and frequency of treatment. Groups generally meet once a week, although in inpatient settings sessions may occur daily. In some studies, groups are time-limited—for example, 12 weekly sessions—whereas in other studies they continue for a year or more.

e) Adverse effects. Acute distress from exposure to emotionally arousing group issues has been reported. Other potential risks of treating patients with borderline personality disorder in group settings include shared resistance to therapeutic work, hostile or other destructive interactions among patients, intensification of transference problems, and symptom "contagion."

f) Implementation issues. Groups take considerable effort to set up and require a group of patients with similar problems and willingness to participate in group treatment. Patients in group therapy must agree to confidentiality regarding the information shared by other patients and to clear guidelines regarding contact with other members outside the group setting. It is critical that there be no "secrets" and that all interactions among group members be discussed in the group, especially information regarding threats of harm to self or others.

4. Couples therapy

a) Goals. The usual goal of couples therapy is to stabilize and strengthen the relationship between the partners or to clarify the nonviability of the relationship. An alternative or additional goal for some is to educate and clarify for the spouse or partner of the patient with borderline personality disorder the process that is taking place within the relationship. Partners of patients with borderline personality disorder may struggle to accommodate the patient's alternating patterns of idealization and depreciation as well as other interpersonal behaviors. As a result, spouses may become dysphoric and self-doubting; they may also become overly attentive and exhibit reaction formation. The goal of treatment is to explore and change these maladaptive reactions and problematic interactions between partners.

b) Efficacy. The literature on the effectiveness of couples therapy for patients with borderline personality disorder is limited to clinical experience and case reports. In some cases, the psychopathology and potential mutual interdependence of each partner may serve a homeostatic function (164–166). Improvement can occur in the relationship when there is recognition of the psychological deficits of both parties. The therapeutic task is to provide an environment in which each spouse can develop self-awareness within the context of the relationship.

c) Adverse effects. One report (41) described an escalation of symptoms when traditional marital therapy was used with a couple who both were diagnosed with borderline personality disorder. Clinical experience would indicate the need for careful psychiatric evaluation of the spouse. When severe character pathology is present in both, the clinician will need to use a multidimensional approach, providing a holding environment for both partners while working toward individuation and intrapsychic growth. Because the spouse's own interpersonal needs or behavioral patterns may, however pathological, serve a homeostatic function within the marriage, couples therapy has the potential to further destabilize the relationship.

d) Implementation issues. At times, it might be helpful for the primary clinician to meet with the spouse or partner and evaluate his or her strengths and weaknesses. It is important to recognize the contingencies of the extent of the partner's loyalty and his or her understanding of what can be expected from the patient with borderline personality disorder before recommending couples therapy. Couples therapy with patients with borderline personality disorder requires considerable understanding of borderline personality disorder and the attendant problems and compensations that such individuals bring to relationships.

5. Family therapy

a) Goals. Relationships in the families of patients with borderline personality disorder are often turbulent and chaotic. The goal of family therapy is to increase family members' understanding of borderline personality disorder, improve relationships between the patient and family members, and enhance the overall functioning of the family.

b) Efficacy.   The published literature on family therapy with patients with borderline personality disorder consists of case reports (167–170) and one published study (12) that found a psychoeducational approach could improve communication, diminish alienation and burden, and diminish conflicts over separation and independence. The clinical literature suggests that family therapy may be useful for some patients—in particular, those who are still dependent on or significantly involved with their families. Some clinicians report the efficacy of dynamically based therapy, whereas others support the efficacy of a psychoeducational approach in which the focus is on educating the family about the diagnosis, improving communication, diminishing hostility and guilt, and diminishing the burden of the illness.

c) Adverse effects.   Some clinicians report that traditional dynamically based family therapy has the potential to end prematurely and have a poor outcome, since patients may alienate their family members or leave the treatment themselves because they feel misunderstood (171) when family involvement is indicated. A psychoeducational approach appears to be less likely to have such adverse effects; however, even psychoeducational approaches can upset family members who wish to avoid knowledge about the illness or involvement in the family member's treatment.

d) Implementation issues.   Traditional dynamically based family therapy requires considerable training and sufficient experience with patients with borderline personality disorder to appreciate their problems and conflicts and to be judicious in the selection of appropriate families.

C. REVIEW OF PHARMACOTHERAPY AND OTHER SOMATIC TREATMENTS

1. SSRI antidepressants

a) Goals.   In borderline personality disorder, SSRIs are used to treat symptoms of affective dysregulation and impulsive-behavioral dyscontrol, particularly depressed mood, anger, and impulsive aggression, including self-mutilation.

b) Efficacy.   Early case reports and small open-label trials with fluoxetine, sertraline, and venlafaxine (a mixed norepinephrine/serotonin reuptake blocker) indicated significant efficacy for symptoms of affective dysregulation, impulsive-behavioral dyscontrol, and cognitive-perceptual difficulties in patients with borderline personality disorder (44–49, 67). Aggression, irritability, depressed mood, and self-mutilation responded to fluoxetine (up to 80 mg/day), venlafaxine (up to 400 mg/day), or sertraline (up to 200 mg/day) in trials of 8–12 weeks (45). An unexpected finding in some of these early reports was that improvement in impulsive behavior appeared rapidly, often within the first week of treatment, and disappeared as quickly with discontinuation or nonadherence. Improvement in impulsive aggression appeared to be independent of effects on depression and anxiety and occurred whether or not the patient had comorbid major depressive disorder (67). Nonresponse to one SSRI did not predict poor response to all SSRIs. For example, some patients who did not respond to fluoxetine, 80 mg/day, responded to a subsequent trial of sertraline. Similarly, patients who did not respond to sertraline, paroxetine, or fluoxetine subsequently responded to venlafaxine. In one study, higher doses and a longer trial (24 weeks) with sertraline converted half of sertraline nonresponders to responders (45).

Three double-blind, placebo-controlled studies have been conducted. Salzman and colleagues (44) conducted a 12-week trial of fluoxetine (20–60 mg/day) in 27 relatively high-functioning subjects (mean Global Assessment Scale score of 74) with borderline personality disorder or borderline traits. Other axis I or axis II comorbid diagnoses were absent, as were recent suicidal behavior, self-mutilation, substance abuse, and current severe aggressive behavior (i.e., behaviors typical of patients with borderline personality disorder seeking treatment). This strategy diminishes generalizability to more seriously ill patients but has the advantage of allowing for a test of efficacy in the absence of comorbidity. For the 22 subjects who completed the study (13 given fluoxetine and nine who received placebo), significant reduction in symptoms of anger and depression and improvement in global functioning were reported for subjects given fluoxetine compared with those given placebo. Improvement in anger was independent of improvement in depressed mood. Improvement was modest, with no subject improving more than 20% on any measure. In addition, a large placebo response was noted.

Markovitz (45) studied 17 patients (nine given fluoxetine, 80 mg/day, and eight given placebo) for 14 weeks. This patient group was noteworthy for the high rate of comorbid axis I mood disorders (10 with major depression, six with bipolar disorder), anxiety disorders, and somatic complaints (e.g., headaches, premenstrual syndrome, irritable bowel syndrome). While this group is more typical of an impaired borderline personality disorder patient population, comorbidity with affective and anxiety disorders confounds interpretation of results. Patients receiving fluoxetine improved significantly more than those given placebo in depression, anxiety, and global symptoms. Measures of impulsive aggression were not included in this study. Some patients with premenstrual syndrome and headaches noted improvement in these somatic presentations with fluoxetine, whereas none improved with placebo.

A double-blind, placebo-controlled study by Coccaro and Kavoussi (67) focused attention on impulsive aggression as a dimensional construct (i.e., a symptom domain found across personality disorders but especially characteristic of borderline personality disorder). Forty subjects with prominent impulsive aggression in the context of a personality disorder, one-third of whom had borderline personality disorder, participated. There was a high rate of comorbidity with dysthymic disorder or depressive disorder not otherwise specified; subjects with major depression and bipolar disorder were excluded. Anxiety disorders, as well as alcohol and drug abuse, were common. In this 12-week, double-blind, placebo-controlled trial, fluoxetine (20–60 mg/day) was more effective than placebo for treatment of verbal aggression and aggression against objects. Improvement was significant by week 10, with improvement in irritability appearing by week 6. Global improvement, favoring fluoxetine, was significant by week 4. As in the open-label trials and the aforementioned Salzman et al. study (44), these investigators found that the effects on aggression and irritability did not appear as a result of improvement in mood or anxiety symptoms.

In summary, these three randomized, double-blind, placebo-controlled studies show efficacy for fluoxetine for affective symptoms—specifically, depressed mood (44, 45), anger (44), and anxiety (45, 67)—although effects on anger and depressed mood appear quantitatively modest. Efficacy has also been demonstrated for impulsive-behavioral symptoms—specifically, verbal and indirect aggression (67)—and global symptom severity (44, 45, 67). Effects on impulsive aggression (67) and anger (44) were independent of effects on affective symptoms, including depressed mood (44, 67) and anxiety (67). Although the three published double-blind, placebo-controlled trials used fluoxetine, open-label studies and clinical experience suggest potential usefulness for other SSRIs.

c) Side effects. The side effect profile of the SSRIs is favorable compared with that of older tricyclic, heterocyclic, or MAOI antidepressants, including low risk in overdose. Side effects reported in these studies are consistent with routine clinical usage.

d) Implementation issues. The SSRI antidepressants may be used in their customary antidepressant dose ranges and durations (e.g., fluoxetine, 20–80 mg/day; sertraline, 100–200 mg/day). One investigator used very high doses of sertraline (200–600 mg/day) for nonresponders, with some improved efficacy (45). At these high doses, peripheral tremor was noted. There are no published studies of continuation and maintenance strategies with SSRIs, although anecdotal reports suggest continuation of improvement in impulsive aggression and self-mutilation for up to several years while the medication is taken and rapid return of symptoms upon discontinuation (49, 172, 173). The duration of treatment is therefore a clinical judgment that depends on the patient's clinical status and medication tolerance at any point in time.

2. Tricyclic and heterocyclic antidepressants

a) Goals. In borderline personality disorder, antidepressants are used for affective dysregulation, manifested most commonly by depressed mood, irritability, and mood lability. Evaluation of antidepressant trials in the treatment of borderline personality disorder must take into account the presence of comorbid axis I mood disorders, which are common in patients with borderline personality disorder. Studies in which there is a preponderance of comorbid axis I depression would be expected to demonstrate a favorable response to antidepressant treatments but may not reflect the pharmacological responsiveness of borderline personality disorder.

b) Efficacy. Double-blind, placebo-controlled trials of tricyclic antidepressants in borderline personality disorder have used amitriptyline, imipramine, and desipramine in both inpatient and outpatient settings. Mianserin, a tetracyclic antidepressant not available in the United States, has been used in an outpatient setting. Most of these studies were parallel comparisons with another medication and placebo. A 5-week inpatient study of patients with borderline personality disorder that compared amitriptyline (mean dose=149 mg/day) with haloperidol and placebo found that amitriptyline decreased depressive symptoms and indirect hostility and enhanced attitudes about self-control compared with placebo (51). It is interesting to note that amitriptyline was not effective for the "core" depressive features of the Hamilton Depression Rating Scale but rather was effective for the seven "associated" symptoms of diurnal variation, depersonalization, paranoid symptoms, obsessive-compulsive symptoms, helplessness, hopelessness, and worthlessness. Patients who had major depression were not more likely to respond. Schizotypal symptoms and paranoia predicted a poor response to amitriptyline.

A small crossover study comparing desipramine (mean dose=162.5 mg/day) with lithium carbonate (mean dose=985.7 mg/day) and placebo in outpatients with borderline personality disorder and minimal axis I mood comorbidity found no significant differences between desipramine and placebo in improvement of affective symptoms, anger, or suicidal symptoms or in therapist or patient perceptions of improvement after 3 and 6 weeks (61).

A small open-label study that assessed the use of amoxapine (an antidepressant with neuroleptic properties) in patients with borderline personality disorder with or without schizotypal personality disorder found that it was not effective for patients with only borderline personality disorder (174). However, it was effective for patients with borderline personality disorder and comorbid schizotypal personality disorder, who had more severe symptoms. This latter group had improvement in cognitive-perceptual, depressive, and global symptoms (174).

In outpatients with a primary diagnosis of atypical depression (which required a current diagnosis of major, minor, or intermittent depression plus associated atypical features) and borderline personality disorder as a secondary diagnosis, imipramine (200 mg/day) produced global improvement in 35% of patients with comorbid borderline personality disorder. In contrast, phenelzine had a 92% response rate in the same sample (57). The presence of borderline personality disorder symptoms predicted a negative global response to imipramine but a positive global response to phenelzine.

One longer-term study was conducted in patients hospitalized for a suicide attempt who were diagnosed with borderline personality disorder or histrionic personality disorder but not axis I depression (175). In this 6-month, double-blind, placebo-controlled study of a low dose of mianserin (30 mg/day), no antidepressant or prophylactic efficacy was found for mianserin compared with placebo for mood symptoms or recurrence of suicidal acts. (The same investigators did demonstrate efficacy against recurrent suicidal acts in this high-risk population with a depot neuroleptic, flupenthixol [80].)

These data suggest that the utility of tricyclic antidepressants in patients with borderline personality disorder is highly questionable. When a clear diagnosis of comorbid major depression can be made, SSRIs are the treatment of choice. When atypical depression is present, the MAOIs have demonstrated superior efficacy to tricyclic antidepressants; however, they must be used with great caution given the high risk of toxicity. (Although the SSRIs have not been extensively studied in atypical depression, at least one double-blind study has indicated comparable efficacy for fluoxetine and phenelzine for the treatment of atypical depression [176].) The efficacy of SSRIs in borderline personality disorder and their favorable safety profile argue for their empirical use in patients with borderline personality disorder with atypical depression.

At best, the response to tricyclic antidepressants (e.g., imipramine) in patients with borderline personality disorder appears modest. The possibility of behavioral toxicity and the known lethality of tricyclic antidepressants in overdose support the preferential use of an SSRI or related antidepressant for patients with borderline personality disorder.

c) Side effects. Common side effects of tricyclic antidepressants include sedation, constipation, dry mouth, and weight gain. The toxicity of tricyclic antidepressants in overdose, including death, indicates that they should be used with caution in patients at risk for suicide. Patients with cardiac conduction abnormalities may experience a fatal arrhythmia with tricyclic antidepressant treatment. For some inpatients with borderline personality disorder, treatment with amitriptyline has paradoxically been associated with behavioral toxicity, consisting of increased suicide threats, paranoid ideation, demanding and assaultive behaviors, and an apparent disinhibition of impulsive behavior (50, 177).

d) Implementation issues.   Other antidepressants are generally preferred over the tricyclic antidepressants for patients with borderline personality disorder. If tricyclic antidepressants are used, the patient should be carefully monitored for signs of toxicity and paradoxical worsening. Doses used in published studies were in the range of 150–250 mg/day of amitriptyline, imipramine, or desipramine. Blood levels may be a useful guide to whether the dose is adequate or toxicity is present.

3. MAOI antidepressants

a) Goals.   MAOIs are used to treat affective symptoms, hostility, and impulsivity related to mood symptoms in patients with borderline personality disorder.

b) Efficacy.   MAOIs have been studied in patients with borderline personality disorder in three placebo-controlled acute treatment trials (55–57). In an outpatient study of phenelzine versus imipramine that selected patients with atypical depression (with borderline personality disorder as a secondary comorbid condition), global improvement occurred in 92% of patients given 60 mg/day of phenelzine compared with 35% of patients given 200 mg/day of imipramine (57). In a study of tranylcypromine, trifluoperazine, alprazolam, and carbamazepine in which borderline personality disorder was a primary diagnosis but comorbid with hysteroid dysphoria (55), tranylcypromine (40 mg/day) improved a broad spectrum of mood symptoms, including depression, anger, rejection sensitivity, and capacity for pleasure. Cowdry and Gardner (55) noted that, "the MAOI proved to be the most effective psychopharmacological agent overall, with clear effects on mood and less prominent effects on behavioral control." Tranylcypromine also significantly decreased impulsivity and suicidality, with a near significant effect on behavioral dyscontrol. When borderline personality disorder is the primary diagnosis, with no selection for atypical depression or hysteroid dysphoria, results are clearly less favorable. Soloff and colleagues (56) studied borderline personality disorder inpatients with comorbid major depression (53%), hysteroid dysphoria (44%), and atypical depression (46%); the patient group was not selected for presence of a depressive disorder. Phenelzine was effective for self-rated anger and hostility but had no specific efficacy, compared with placebo or haloperidol, for atypical depression or hysteroid dysphoria. These three acute trials were 5–6 weeks in duration. A 16-week continuation study of the responding patients in a follow-up study (68) showed some continuing modest improvement over placebo beyond the acute 5-week trial for depression and irritability. Phenelzine appeared to be activating, which was considered favorable in the clinical setting.

On balance, these studies suggest that MAOIs are often helpful for atypical depressive symptoms, anger, hostility, and impulsivity in patients with borderline personality disorder. These effects appear to be independent of a current mood disorder diagnosis (56), although one study found a nonsignificantly higher rate of MAOI response for patients with a past history of major depression or bipolar II disorder (55).

c) Side effects.   Phenelzine can cause weight gain (56) and can be difficult to tolerate. Other side effects include orthostatic hypotension (55). Fatal hypertensive crises are the most serious potential side effect of MAOIs, although no study reported any hypertensive crises due to violation of the tyramine dietary restriction. The initial clinical picture of MAOI poisoning is one of agitation, delirium, hallucinations, hyperreflexia, tachycardia, tachypnea, dilated pupils, diaphoresis, and, often, convulsions. Hyperpyrexia is one of the most serious problems (178).

d) Implementation issues. Doses of phenelzine and tranylcypromine used in published studies ranged from 60–90 mg/day and 10–60 mg/day, respectively. Experienced clinicians may vary doses according to their usual practice in treating depressive or anxiety disorders. Adherence to a tyramine-free diet is critically important and requires careful patient instruction, ideally supplemented by a printed guide to tyramine-rich foods and medication interactions, especially over-the-counter decongestants found in common cold and allergy remedies. Given the impulsivity of patients with borderline personality disorder, it is helpful to review in detail the potential for serious medical consequences of nonadherence to dietary restrictions, the symptoms of hypertensive crisis, and an emergency treatment plan in case of a hypertensive crisis. Patients must be instructed to discontinue an SSRI long enough in advance of instituting MAOI therapy to avoid precipitating a serotonin syndrome.

4. Lithium carbonate and anticonvulsant mood stabilizers

a) Goals. Lithium carbonate and the anticonvulsant mood stabilizers carbamazepine and divalproex sodium are used to treat symptoms of behavioral dyscontrol in borderline personality disorder, with possible efficacy for symptoms of affective dysregulation.

b) Efficacy. The efficacy of lithium carbonate for bipolar disorder led to treatment trials in patients with personality disorders characterized by mood dysregulation and impulsive aggression. Rifkin and colleagues (179, 180) demonstrated improvement in mood swings in 21 patients with emotionally unstable character disorder, a DSM-I diagnosis characterized by brief but nonreactive mood swings, both depressive and hypomanic, in the context of a chronically maladaptive personality resembling "hysterical character." In this placebo-controlled crossover study (each medication was taken for 6 weeks), there was decreased variation in mood (i.e., fewer "mood swings") and global improvement in 14 of 21 patients during lithium treatment. Subsequent case reports demonstrated that lithium had mood-stabilizing and antiaggressive effects in patients with borderline personality disorder (181, 182).

One double-blind, placebo-controlled crossover study compared lithium with desipramine in 17 patients with borderline personality disorder (61). All patients took lithium for 6 weeks (mean dose=985.7 mg/day) and received concurrent psychotherapy. Among 10 patients completing both lithium and placebo treatments, therapists' blind ratings indicated greater improvement during the lithium trial, although patients' self-ratings did not reflect significant differences between lithium and placebo. The authors noted that therapists were favorably impressed by decreases in impulsivity during the lithium trial, an improvement not fully appreciated by the patients themselves. There has never been a double-blind, placebo-controlled trial of the antiaggressive effects of lithium carbonate in patients with borderline personality disorder selected for histories of impulsive aggression.

The anticonvulsant mood stabilizer carbamazepine has been studied in two double-blind, placebo-controlled studies that used very different patient groups, resulting in inconsistent findings. Gardner and Cowdry (55, 62), in a crossover trial, studied female outpatients with borderline personality disorder and comorbid hysteroid dysphoria along with extensive histories of behavioral dyscontrol. Patients underwent a 6-week trial of carbamazepine (mean dose=820 mg/day) and continued receiving psychotherapy. Patients had decreased frequency and severity of behavioral dyscontrol during the carbamazepine trial. Among all patients, there were significantly fewer suicide attempts or other major dyscontrol episodes along with improvement in anxiety, anger, and euphoria (by a physician's assessment only) with carbamazepine treatment compared with placebo.

De la Fuente and Lotstra (63) failed to replicate these findings, although this may be due to their small study group size (N=20). These investigators conducted a double-blind, placebo-controlled trial of carbamazepine in inpatients with a primary diagnosis of borderline personality disorder. Patients with any comorbid axis I disorder, a history of epilepsy, or EEG abnormalities were excluded. Unlike in the Cowdry and Gardner study (55), patients were not selected for histories of behavioral dyscontrol. There were no significant differences between carbamazepine and placebo on measures of affective or cognitive-perceptual symptoms, impulsive-behavioral "acting out," or global symptoms.

Divalproex sodium has been used in open-label trials targeting the agitation and aggression of patients with borderline personality disorder in a state hospital setting (70) and mood instability and impulsivity in an outpatient clinic (66). Wilcox (70) reported a 68% decrease in time spent in seclusion as well as improvement in anxiety, tension, and global symptoms among 30 patients with borderline personality disorder receiving divalproex sodium (with dose titrated to a level of 100 mg/ml) for 6 weeks in a state hospital. Patients did not have "psychiatric comorbid conditions" (by clinical assessment), although five had an EEG abnormality (but no seizure disorders); concurrent psychotropic medications were allowed. An abnormal EEG predicted improvement with divalproex sodium. The author noted that both the antiaggressive and antianxiety effects of divalproex sodium appeared instrumental in decreasing agitation and time spent in seclusion.

An open-label study by Stein and colleagues (66) enrolled 11 cooperative outpatients with borderline personality disorder, all of whom had been in psychotherapy for a minimum of 8 weeks and were free of other medications before starting divalproex sodium treatment, which was titrated to levels of 50–100 mg/ml. Among the eight patients who completed the study, four responded in terms of global improvement and observed irritability; physician ratings of mood, anxiety, anger, impulsivity, and rejection sensitivity; and patient ratings of global improvement. There were no significant changes in measures specific for depression and anxiety, but baseline depression and anxiety scores were low in this population.

Kavoussi and Coccaro (69) also reported significant improvement in impulsive aggression and irritability after 4 weeks of treatment with divalproex sodium in 10 patients with impulsive aggression in the context of a cluster B personality disorder, five of whom (four completers) had borderline personality disorder. Among the eight patients who completed the 8-week trial, six had a 50% or greater reduction in aggression and irritability. All patients had not responded to a previous trial with fluoxetine (up to 60 mg/day for 8 weeks).

Only one small, randomized controlled trial of divalproex has been reported that involved patients with borderline personality disorder (65). Among 12 patients randomly assigned to divalproex, only six completed a 10-week trial, five of whom responded in terms of global measures. There was improvement in depression, albeit not statistically significant, and aggression was unchanged. None of the four patients randomly assigned to placebo completed the study.

In summary, preliminary evidence suggests that lithium carbonate and the mood stabilizers carbamazepine and divalproex may be useful in treating behavioral dyscontrol and affective dysregulation in some patients with borderline personality disorder, although further studies are needed. The only report on the newer anticonvulsants (i.e., gabapentin, lamotrigine, topiramate) in borderline personality disorder is a case series in which three of eight patients had a good response to lamotrigine (183). Because of the paucity of evidence concerning these agents, careful consideration of the risks and benefits is recommended when using such medications pending the publication of findings from systematic studies.

c) Side effects. Although lithium commonly causes side effects, most are minor or can be reduced or eliminated by lowering the dose or changing the dosage schedule. More common side effects include polyuria, polydipsia, weight gain, cognitive problems (e.g., dulling, poor concentration), tremor, sedation or lethargy, and gastrointestinal distress (e.g., nausea). Lithium may also have renal effects and may cause hypothyroidism. Lithium is potentially fatal in overdose and should be used with caution in patients at risk of suicide.

Carbamazepine's most common side effects include neurological symptoms (e.g., diplopia), blurred vision, fatigue, nausea, and ataxia. Other side effects include skin rash, mild leukopenia or thrombocytopenia, and hyponatremia. Rare, idiosyncratic, but potentially fatal side effects include agranulocytosis, aplastic anemia, hepatic failure, exfoliative dermatitis, and pancreatitis. Carbamazepine may be fatal in overdose. In studies of patients with borderline personality disorder, carbamazepine has been reported to cause melancholic depression (64).

Common dose-related side effects of valproate include gastrointestinal distress (e.g., nausea), benign hepatic transaminase elevations, tremor, sedation, and weight gain. With long-term use, women may be at risk of developing polycystic ovaries or hyperandrogenism. Mild, asymptomatic leukopenia and thrombocytopenia occur less frequently. Rare, idiosyncratic, but potentially fatal adverse events include hepatic failure, pancreatitis, and agranulocytosis.

d) Implementation issues. Full guidelines for the use of these medications can be found in the APA *Practice Guideline for the Treatment of Patients With Bipolar Disorder* (85). Lithium carbonate and the anticonvulsant mood stabilizers are used in their full therapeutic doses, with plasma levels guiding dosing. Routine precautions observed for the use of these medications in other disorders also apply to their use in borderline personality disorder, e.g., plasma level monitoring of thyroid and kidney function with prolonged lithium use, periodic measure of WBC count with carbamazepine therapy, and hematological and liver function tests for divalproex sodium.

5. Anxiolytic agents

a) Goals. Anxiolytic medications are used to treat the many manifestations of anxiety in patients with borderline personality disorder, both as an acute and as a chronic symptom.

b) Efficacy. Despite widespread use, there is a paucity of studies investigating the use of anxiolytic medications in borderline personality disorder. Cowdry and Gardner (55) included alprazolam in their double-blind, placebo-controlled, crossover study of outpatients with borderline personality disorder, comorbid hysteroid dysphoria, and extensive histories of behavioral dyscontrol. Use of alprazolam (mean dose=4.7 mg/day) was associated with greater suicidality and episodes of serious behavioral dyscontrol (drug overdoses, self-mutilation, and throwing a chair at a child). This occurred in seven (58%) of 12 patients taking alprazolam compared with one (8%) of 13 patients receiving placebo. However, in a small number of patients (N=3), alprazolam was noted to be helpful for anxiety in carefully selected patients with borderline personality disorder (52). Case reports suggest that clonazepam is helpful as an adjunctive agent in the treatment of impulsivity, violent outbursts, and anxiety in a variety of disorders, including borderline personality disorder (54).

Although clinicians have presented preliminary experiences with nonbenzodiazepine anxiolytics in patients with borderline personality disorder (e.g., buspirone) (184), there are currently no published studies of these anxiolytics in borderline personality disorder.

c) Side effects. Behavioral disinhibition, resulting in impulsive and assaultive behaviors, has been reported with alprazolam in patients with borderline personality disorder. Benzodiazepines, in general, should be used with care because of the potential for abuse and the development of pharmacological tolerance with prolonged use. These are particular risks in patients with a history of substance use.

d) Implementation issues. In the absence of clear evidence-based recommendations, dose and duration of treatment must be guided by clinical need and judgment, keeping in mind the potential for abuse and pharmacological tolerance.

6. Opiate antagonists

a) Goals. It has been suggested that the relative subjective numbing and physical analgesia that patients with borderline personality disorder often feel during episodes of self-mutilation, as well as the reported sense of relative well-being afterward, might be due to release of endogenous opiates (185–187). Opiate antagonists have been employed in an attempt to block mutilation-induced analgesia and euphoria and thereby reduce self-injurious behavior in patients with borderline personality disorder.

b) Efficacy. Clinical case reports (188) and several small case series have assessed the efficacy of opiate antagonists for self-injurious behavior, and two suggested some improvement in this behavior (189, 190). One small, double-blind study involving female patients with borderline personality disorder with a history of self-injurious behavior who underwent a stress challenge showed no effect of opiate receptor blockade with naloxone on cold pressor pain perception or mood ratings (191). While the stress level may not have been high enough to mimic clinical situations, the study does not support the theory that opiate antagonism plays a role in reducing self-injurious behavior.

Despite the few promising clinical case reports, these reports are very preliminary, and there is no clear evidence from well-controlled trials indicating that opiate antagonists are effective in reducing self-injurious behavior among patients with borderline personality disorder.

c) Side effects. Nausea and diarrhea are occasionally reported (190).

d) Implementation issues. In published reports, the typical dose of naltrexone was 50 mg/day. No time limit for treatment emerges from the literature, but the effect is presumably reversed when the medication stops.

7. Neuroleptics

a) Goals. The primary goal of treatment with neuroleptics in borderline personality disorder is to reduce acute symptom severity in all symptom domains, particularly schizotypal symptoms, psychosis, anger, and hostility.

b) Efficacy. Early clinical experience with neuroleptics targeted the "micropsychotic" or schizotypal symptoms of borderline personality disorder. However, affective symptoms (mood, anxiety, anger) and somatic complaints also improved with low doses of haloperidol, perphenazine, and thiothixene. An open-label trial of thioridazine (mean dose=92 mg/day) led to marked improvement in impulsive-behavioral symptoms, global symptom severity, and overall borderline psychopathology (78). Similar findings were reported for adolescents with borderline personality disorder treated with flupentixol (mean dose=3 mg/day) (77), with improvement in impulsivity, depression, and global functioning.

Systematic, parallel studies that compared neuroleptics without a placebo control condition also reported a broad spectrum of efficacy. Leone (73) found that loxapine succinate (mean dose=14.5 mg/day) or chlorpromazine (mean dose=110 mg/day) improved depressed mood, anxiety, anger/hostility, and suspiciousness. Serban and Siegel (74) reported that thiothixene (mean dose=9.4 mg/day, SD=7.6) or haloperidol (mean dose=3.0 mg/day, SD=0.8) produced improvement in anxiety, depression, derealization, paranoia (ideas of reference), general symptoms, and a global measure of borderline psychopathology.

Subsequent double-blind, placebo-controlled trials also suggested a broad spectrum of efficacy for low-dose neuroleptics in the treatment of borderline personality disorder. Acute symptom severity improved in cognitive-perceptual, affective, and impulsive-behavioral symptom domains, although efficacy for schizotypal symptoms, psychoticism, anger, and hostility were most consistently noted.

Many of the double-blind, placebo-controlled studies of neuroleptics in borderline personality disorder are noteworthy for biases in sample selection that strongly affected outcomes. In a study of patients with borderline or schizotypal personality disorder and at least one psychotic symptom (which biased the sample toward cognitive-perceptual symptoms), thiothixene (mean dose=8.7 mg/day for up to 12 weeks) was more effective than placebo for psychotic cluster symptoms—specifically illusions and ideas of reference—and self-rated obsessive-compulsive and phobic anxiety symptoms but not depression or global functioning (75). The more severely symptomatic patients were at baseline (e.g., in terms of illusions, ideas of reference, or obsessive-compulsive and phobic anxiety symptoms), the better they responded to thiothixene (75).

Cowdry and Gardner (55) conducted a complex, placebo-controlled, four-drug crossover study in borderline personality disorder outpatients with trifluoperazine (mean dose=7.8 mg/day). Patients were required to meet criteria for hysteroid dysphoria and have a history of extensive behavioral dyscontrol, introducing a bias toward affective and impulsive-behavioral symptoms. All patients were receiving psychotherapy. Those patients who were able to keep taking trifluoperazine for 3 weeks or longer (seven of 12 patients) had improved mood, with significant improvement over placebo on physician ratings of depression, anxiety, rejection sensitivity, and suicidality.

Soloff and colleagues (50, 51) studied acutely ill inpatients, comparing haloperidol with amitriptyline and placebo in a 5-week trial. Patients who received haloperidol (mean dose=4.8 mg/day) improved significantly more than those receiving placebo across all symptom domains (50), including global measures, self- and observer-rated depression, anger and hostility, schizotypal symptoms, psychoticism, and impulsive behaviors (51). Haloperidol was as effective as amitriptyline for depressive symptoms.

However, a second study by the same group (56) that used the same design but compared haloperidol with phenelzine and placebo failed to replicate the broad-spectrum efficacy of haloperidol (mean dose=3.9 mg/day). Efficacy for haloperidol was limited to hostile belligerence and impulsive-aggressive behaviors, and placebo effects were powerful. Patients in this study had milder symptoms, especially in the cognitive-perceptual and impulsive-behavioral symptom domains, than patients in the first study.

Cornelius and colleagues (68) followed a subset of the aforementioned group who had responded to haloperidol, phenelzine, or placebo for 16 weeks following acute treatment. Patients' intolerance of the medication, a high dropout rate, and non-adherence were decisive factors in this study. The attrition rates at 22 weeks were 87.5% for haloperidol, 65.7% for phenelzine, and 58.1% for placebo. Further significant improvement with haloperidol treatment (compared with placebo) occurred only for irritability (with improvement for hostility that was not statistically significant). Depressive symptoms significantly worsened with haloperidol treatment over time, which was attributed, in part, to the side effect of akinesia. Clinical improvement was modest and of limited clinical importance.

Montgomery and Montgomery (80) controlled for nonadherence by using depot flupenthixol decanoate, 20 mg once a month, in a continuation study of recurrently parasuicidal patients with borderline personality disorder and histrionic personality disorder. Over a 6-month period, patients receiving flupentixol had a significant decrease in suicidal behaviors compared with the placebo group. Significant differences emerged by the fourth month and were sustained through 6 months of treatment. This important study awaits replication.

The introduction of the newer atypical neuroleptics increases clinicians' options for treating borderline personality disorder. To date, findings from only two small open-label trials have been published, both with clozapine. Frankenburg and Zanarini (81) reported that clozapine (mean dose=253.3 mg/day, SD=163.7) improved positive and negative psychotic symptoms and global functioning (but not depression or other symptoms) in 15 patients with borderline personality disorder and comorbid axis I psychotic disorder not otherwise specified who had not responded to (or were intolerant of) other neuroleptics. Improvement was modest but statistically significant. Patients were recruited from a larger study of patients with treatment-resistant psychotic disorders, raising the question of whether their psychotic symptoms were truly part of their borderline personality disorder.

These concerns were addressed by Benedetti and colleagues (71), who excluded all patients with axis I psychotic disorders from their cohort of patients with refractory borderline personality disorder. Target symptoms included "psychotic-like" symptoms that are more typical of borderline personality disorder. Patients had not responded to at least 4 months of prior treatment with medication and psychotherapy. In a 4-month, open-label trial of 12 patients treated with clozapine (mean dose=

43.8 mg/day, SD=18.8) and concurrent psychotherapy, a low dose of clozapine improved symptoms in all domains—cognitive-perceptual, affective, and impulsive-behavioral.

Despite a lack of data, clinicians are increasingly using olanzapine, risperidone, and quetiapine for patients with borderline personality disorder. These medications have less risk than clozapine and may be better tolerated than the typical neuroleptics. Schulz and colleagues (83) presented preliminary data from a double-blind, placebo-controlled, 8-week trial of risperidone in 27 patients with borderline personality disorder who received an average dose of 2.5 mg/day (to a maximum of 4 mg/day). On global measures of functioning, there was no significant difference between risperidone and placebo, although the authors noted that risperidone-treated patients were "diverging from the placebo group" in paranoia, psychoticism, interpersonal sensitivity, and phobic anxiety (83). The same group conducted an 8-week, open-label study of olanzapine in patients with borderline personality disorder and comorbid dysthymia (82). Patients received an average dose of 7.5 mg/day (range=2.5–10 mg/day). Among the 11 completers, significant improvement was reported across all domains, with particular improvement noted in depression, interpersonal sensitivity, psychoticism, anxiety, and anger/hostility. These medications require further investigation in double-blind studies.

In summary, neuroleptics are the best-studied psychotropic medications for borderline personality disorder. The literature supports the use of low-dose neuroleptics for the acute management of global symptom severity, with specific efficacy for schizotypal symptoms and psychoticism, anger, and hostility. Relief of global symptom severity in the acute setting may be due, in part, to nonspecific "tranquilizer" effects of neuroleptics, whereas symptom-specific actions against psychoticism, anger, and hostility may relate more directly to dopaminergic blockade. Acute treatment effects of neuroleptic drugs in borderline personality disorder tend to be modest but clinically and statistically significant.

Two studies that addressed continuation and maintenance treatment of a patient with borderline personality disorder with neuroleptics had contradictory results. The Montgomery and Montgomery study (80) reported efficacy for recurrent parasuicidal behaviors, whereas the Cornelius et al. study (68) suggested very modest utility for only irritability and hostility. More controlled trials are needed to investigate low-dose neuroleptics in continuation and maintenance treatment.

c) Side effects. Dropout rates in neuroleptic trials in borderline outpatients range from 13.7% for a 6-week trial (73) to 48.3% for a 12-week trial (75) to 87.5% for a 22-week continuation study (68). In acute studies, patient nonadherence is often due to typical medication side effects, e.g., extrapyramidal symptoms, akathisia, sedation, and hypotension. Patients with borderline personality disorder who have experienced relief of acute symptoms with low-dose neuroleptics may not tolerate the side effects of the drug with longer-term treatment. The risk of tardive dyskinesia must be considered in any decision to continue neuroleptic medication over the long term. Thioridazine has been associated with cardiac rhythm disturbances related to widening of the Q-T interval and should be avoided. In the case of clozapine, the risk of agranulocytosis is especially problematic. While the newer atypical neuroleptics promise a more favorable side effect profile, evidence of efficacy in borderline personality disorder is still awaited. Neuroleptics should be given in the context of a supportive doctor-patient relationship in which side effects and nonadherence are addressed frequently.

d) Implementation issues.   All studies have used a low dose and demonstrated beneficial effects within several weeks. With the exception of one study that used a depot neuroleptic (flupentixol, which is not available in the United States), all medications were given orally and daily. Acute treatment studies are a good model for acute clinical care and typically range from 5 to 12 weeks in duration. There is insufficient evidence to make a strong recommendation concerning continuation and maintenance therapies. At present, this is best left to the clinician's judgment after carefully weighing the risks and benefits for the individual patient. CBC monitoring must be done if clozapine is used.

8. ECT

a) Goals.   The goal of ECT in patients with borderline personality disorder is to decrease depressive symptoms in individuals with a comorbid axis I mood disorder, which is present in as many as one-half of hospitalized patients with borderline personality disorder.

b) Efficacy.   Most of the clinical and empirical literature that describes experience with ECT in patients with major depression comorbid with personality disorders does not report results specifically for borderline personality disorder. Although studies that used a naturalistic design have had inconsistent findings, patients with major depression and a comorbid personality disorder were generally less responsive to somatic treatments than patients with major depression alone.

In one naturalistic follow-up study (based on chart review), there was no significant difference in recovery rates for 10 patients with major depressive disorder and a personality disorder (40% recovery) compared with 41 patients with major depressive disorder alone (65.9% recovery) (192). In another study, involving 1,471 depressed inpatients, depressed patients with a personality disorder were 50% less likely to be recovered at hospital discharge than depressed patients without a personality disorder (193).

Several uncontrolled studies found that outcome was dependent on the time of assessment. In one small study (194), there were no significant differences in immediate response to ECT between depressed subjects with or without a personality disorder; however, at a 6-month follow-up evaluation, the patients with a personality disorder had more rehospitalizations and more severe depression symptoms. Conversely, in another uncontrolled study of inpatients with major depression (195), compared with depressed patients without a personality disorder, those with a personality disorder had a poorer outcome in terms of depression and social functioning immediately following treatment. However, after 6 and 12 weeks of follow-up, there were no differences between the two groups in terms of depression and social functioning. The number of rehospitalizations did not differ between groups at the 6-month and 12-month follow-up evaluations.

In another small study (N=16) (196–198) that used the self-rated Millon Clinical Multiaxial Inventory—II and assessed borderline personality disorder, there was significant improvement in avoidant, histrionic, aggressive/sadistic, and schizotypal personality traits with ECT. Improvements were noted in passive-aggressive and borderline personality traits that did not reach statistical significance. The presence of pretreatment borderline traits predicted poorer outcome with ECT (198).

Although the results of these studies appear somewhat divergent, most found that patients with major depression and a personality disorder have a less favorable outcome with ECT than depressed patients without a personality disorder.

c) Adverse effects.   Because ECT is not recommended for borderline personality disorder per se, adverse effects are not described here and can be found in the APA *Practice Guideline for the Treatment of Patients With Major Depressive Disorder* (84).

d) Implementation issues.   The affective dysregulation, low self-esteem, pessimism, chronic suicidality, and self-mutilation of patients with borderline personality disorder are often misconstrued as axis I depression. Clinical experience suggests that, not infrequently, these characterological manifestations of borderline personality disorder are treated with ECT, often resulting in a poor outcome. Although there is a paucity of ECT studies involving patients with borderline personality disorder, a recommendation for ECT in these patients with comorbid major depression should be guided by the presence and severity of verifiable neurovegetative symptoms, e.g., sleep disturbance, appetite disturbance, weight change, low energy, and anhedonia. These symptoms should ideally be confirmed by outside observers, as they provide an objective way to assess treatment response. Perhaps the greatest challenge for the clinician is not when to institute ECT in the depressed patient with borderline personality disorder but when to stop. As the neurovegetative symptoms of major depression resolve, many patients continue to have borderline features that clinical experience suggests are unresponsive to ECT. Knowledge of the patient's personality functioning before the onset of major depression is critical to knowing when the "baseline" has been achieved. Many patients with borderline personality disorder who are considered nonresponsive to ECT because of persistence of depressive features are, in fact, already in remission from their axis I depression but continue to experience chronic characterological depressive features.

Notable progress has been made in our understanding of borderline personality disorder and its treatment. However, there are many remaining questions regarding treatments with demonstrated efficacy, including how to optimally use them to achieve the best health outcomes for patients with borderline personality disorder. In addition, many therapeutic modalities have received little empirical investigation for borderline personality disorder and require further study. The efficacy of various treatments also needs to be studied in populations such as adolescents, the elderly, forensic populations, and patients in long-term institutional settings. The following is a sample of the types of research questions that require further study.

PART C:
FUTURE RESEARCH NEEDS

VII. PSYCHOTHERAPY

Many aspects of psychotherapy in the treatment of borderline personality disorder require further investigation. For example, further controlled treatment studies of psychodynamic psychotherapy, dialectical behavior therapy, and other forms of cognitive behavior therapy are needed, particularly in outpatient settings. In addition, psychotherapeutic interventions that have received less investigation, such as group therapy, couples therapy, and family interventions, require study. The following are some specific questions that need to be addressed by future research:

- What is the relative efficacy of different psychotherapeutic approaches? Which types of patients respond to which types of psychotherapy?
- What components of dialectical behavior therapy and psychodynamic psychotherapy are responsible for their efficacy? What common elements of these treatments are responsible for their efficacy?
- What are the indications for use of psychodynamic psychotherapy and dialectical behavior therapy? How does the presence of certain clinical features (e.g., prominent self-destructive behavior or dissociative features) affect response to these treatments?
- To what extent is a good outcome due to the unique components of these treatments versus the amount of treatment received?
- How effective are psychodynamic psychotherapy and dialectical behavior therapy when used in the community rather than in specialized treatment settings, and how can these treatments be optimally implemented in community settings?
- What is the optimal duration of psychotherapy for patients with borderline personality disorder?
- Is there a model of brief psychotherapy (12–30 sessions) that is effective for borderline personality disorder?
- What are the optimal frequencies of psychotherapeutic contact for different psychotherapies during different stages of treatment?
- What is the relative efficacy of psychotherapy versus pharmacotherapy for patients with borderline personality disorder? Do certain patients respond better to one treatment modality than to the other?
- What is the relative efficacy of a combination of psychotherapy and pharmacotherapy versus either treatment modality alone?

VIII. PHARMACOTHERAPY AND OTHER SOMATIC TREATMENTS

Many aspects of pharmacotherapy in the treatment of borderline personality disorder also require investigation. Further controlled treatment studies of medications—in particular, those that have received relatively little investigation (for example, atypical neuroleptics)—are needed. Studies of continuation and maintenance treatment as well as treatment discontinuation are especially needed, as are systematic studies of treatment sequences and algorithms. The following are some specific questions that need to be addressed by future research:

- What is the relative efficacy of different pharmacological approaches for the behavioral dimensions of borderline personality disorder?
- What is the relative efficacy of different pharmacological augmentation and combination strategies, and what is their efficacy compared with treatment with single agents?
- How does the presence of certain clinical features (for example, prominent self-destructive behavior or dissociative features) affect response to pharmacotherapy?
- What is the minimal dose and duration of an adequate trial for different medications in patients with borderline personality disorder?
- What is the optimal duration of different types of medication treatment?
- What are the indications for discontinuation of effective pharmacological treatment?
- Are atypical neuroleptics or typical neuroleptics more effective or better tolerated in patients with borderline personality disorder?
- How efficacious are mood stabilizers for patients with borderline personality disorder, and which patients are most likely to benefit from this treatment? Are certain mood stabilizers more effective than others?
- What role should ECT have in the treatment of patients with refractory or severe borderline personality disorder?

APPENDIXES:
PSYCHOPHARMACOLOGICAL TREATMENT ALGORITHMS

APPENDIX 1. Psychopharmacological Treatment of Affective Dysregulation Symptoms in Patients With Borderline Personality Disorder[a]

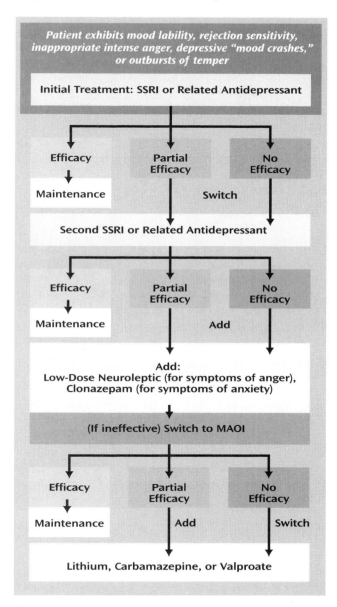

[a]Algorithm based on clinical judgment that uses evidence currently in the literature, following the format of the International Psychopharmacology Algorithm Project (2). The first step in the algorithm is generally supported by the best empirical evidence. Recommendations may not be applicable to all patients or take individual needs into account. The empirical research studies on which these recommendations are based may be "first trials" involving previously untreated patients and may not take into account previous patient nonresponse to one, two, or even three levels of the algorithm (i.e., patients who, by definition, have more refractory disorders). There are no empirical trials of the complete algorithm.

APPENDIX 2. Psychopharmacological Treatment of Impulsive-Behavioral Dyscontrol Symptoms in Patients With Borderline Personality Disorder[a]

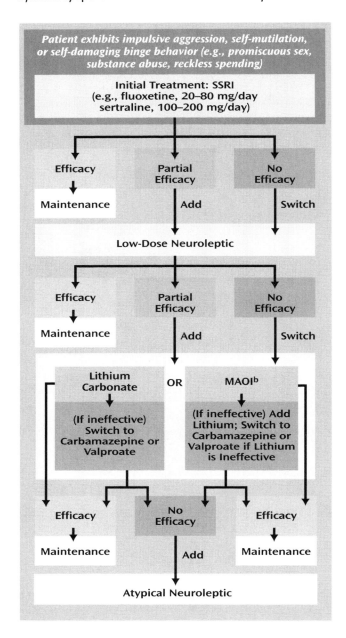

[a]Algorithm based on clinical judgment that uses evidence currently in the literature, following the format of the International Psychopharmacology Algorithm Project (2). The first step in the algorithm is generally supported by the best empirical evidence. Recommendations may not be applicable to all patients or take individual needs into account. The empirical research studies on which these recommendations are based may be "first trials" involving previously untreated patients and may not take into account previous patient nonresponse to one, two, or even three levels of the algorithm (i.e., patients who, by definition, have more refractory disorders). There are no empirical trials of the complete algorithm.

[b]SSRI treatment must be discontinued and followed with an adequate washout period before initiating treatment with an MAOI.

APPENDIX 3. Psychopharmacological Treatment of Cognitive-Perceptual Symptoms in Patients With Borderline Personality Disorder[a]

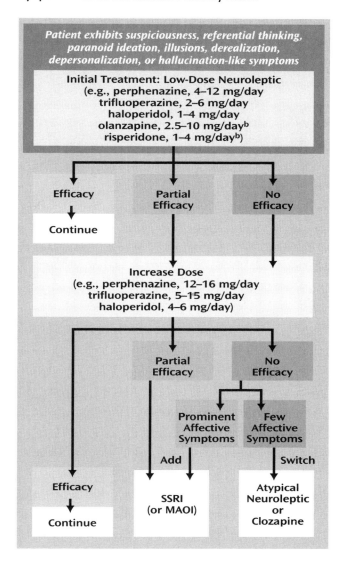

[a]Algorithm based on clinical judgment that uses evidence currently in the literature, following the format of the International Psychopharmacology Algorithm Project (2). The first step in the algorithm is generally supported by the best empirical evidence. Recommendations may not be applicable to all patients or take individual needs into account. The empirical research studies on which these recommendations are based may be "first trials" involving previously untreated patients and may not take into account previous patient nonresponse to one, two, or even three levels of the algorithm (i.e., patients who, by definition, have more refractory disorders). There are no empirical trials of the complete algorithm.

[b]The generally favorable side effect profiles of the newer atypical neuroleptic medications compared with those of conventional neuroleptics underscore the need for careful empirical trials of these newer medications in the treatment of patients with borderline personality disorder.

INDIVIDUALS AND ORGANIZATIONS THAT SUBMITTED COMMENTS

Gerald Adler, M.D.
Hagop Akiskal, M.D.
Deborah Antai-Otong, M.S.,
    R.N., P.M.H.N.P., C.S.
Lorna Benjamin, Ph.D.
Sandra Smith Bjork, R.N., J.D.
Nashaat N. Boutros, M.D.
Daniel Buie, M.D.
Kenneth Busch, M.D.
Carlyle H. Chan, M.D.
Richard D. Chessick, M.D.,
    Ph.D.
Diego Cohen, M.D.
Nancy Collins, R.N., M.P.H.
Alv A. Dahl, M.D.
Dave M. Davis, M.D.
Diana Dell, M.D.
Anita S. Everett, M.D.
Robert Findling, M.D.
Douglas H. Finestone, M.D.
Arnold Goldberg, M.D.
William M. Greenberg, M.D.

Elliot A. Harris, M.D.
Al Herzog, M.D.
Eric Hollander, M.D.
Patricia Hoffman Judd, Ph.D.
Morten Kjolbye, M.D.
Ronald Koegler, M.D.
Paul S. Links, M.D.
Cesare Maffei, M.D.
Paul Markovitz, M.D., Ph.D.
John C. Markowitz, M.D.
James F. Masterson, M.D.
William Meissner, M.D.
Mary D. Moller, M.S.N., C.S.,
    P.M.H.N.P.
Robert Michels, M.D.
Richard Munich, M.D.
Nathan A. Munn, M.D.
Andrei Novac, M.D.
Stefano Pallanti, M.D.
Joel Paris, M.D.
Jane L. Pearson, Ph.D.
Gary Peterson, M.D.

Eric M. Plakun, M.D.
Charles W. Portney, M.D.
Lawrence H. Rockland, M.D.
Barbara Rosenfeld, M.D.
Marc Rothman, M.D.
Marian Scheinholtz, M.S.,
    O.T.R.L.
Judy Sigmund, M.D.
Kenneth R. Silk, M.D.
Andrew E. Skodol, M.D.
Robert Stern, M.D., Ph.D.
Nada L. Stotland, M.D., M.P.H.
Richard T. Suchinsky, M.D.
Peter J. Sukin, M.D.
Arthur Summer, M.D.
Marijo Tamburrino, M.D.
William R. Tatomer, M.D.
Per Vaglum, M.D.
Robert S. Wallerstein, M.D.
Sidney Weissman, M.D.
Drew Westen, Ph.D.
Jerome Winer, M.D.

American Academy of Ophthalmology
American College of Obstetrics and
    Gynecology
American College of Radiology
American Occupational Therapy Association
American Psychiatric Nurses Association
American Psychoanalytic Association
Commonwealth of Virginia Department of
    Mental Health, Mental Retardation and
    Substance Abuse Services

Illinois Psychiatric Society
International Society for the Study of
    Personality Disorders
New Jersey Psychiatric Association
Norwegian Psychiatric Association
Royal Australian and New Zealand College of
    Psychiatrists

REFERENCES

The following coding system is used to indicate the nature of the supporting evidence in the references:

[A] *Randomized clinical trial.* A study of an intervention in which subjects are prospectively followed over time; there are treatment and control groups; subjects are randomly assigned to the two groups; both the subjects and the investigators are blind to the assignments.

[B] *Clinical trial.* A prospective study in which an intervention is made and the results of that intervention are tracked longitudinally; study does not meet standards for a randomized clinical trial.

[C] *Cohort or longitudinal study.* A study in which subjects are prospectively followed over time without any specific intervention.

[D] *Case-control study.* A study in which a group of patients and a group of control subjects are identified in the present and information about them is pursued retrospectively or backward in time.

[E] *Review with secondary data analysis.* A structured analytic review of existing data, e.g., a meta-analysis or a decision analysis.

[F] *Review.* A qualitative review and discussion of previously published literature without a quantitative synthesis of the data.

[G] *Other.* Textbooks, expert opinion, case reports, and other reports not included above.

1. American Psychiatric Association: Diagnostic and Statistical Manual of Mental Disorders, 4th ed, Text Revision (DSM-IV-TR). Washington, DC, APA, 2000 [G]
2. Jobson KO, Potter WZ: International Psychopharmacology Algorithm Project report. Psychopharmacol Bull 1995; 31:457–507 [F]
3. American Psychiatric Association: Practice Guideline for Psychiatric Evaluation of Adults. Am J Psychiatry 1995; 152(Nov suppl) [G]
4. Kernberg OF, Selzer M, Koenigsberg H, Carr A, Appelbaum A: Psychodynamic Psychotherapy of Borderline Patients. New York, Basic Books, 1989 [G]
5. Linehan MM, Heard HL, Armstrong HE: Naturalistic follow-up of a behavioral treatment for chronically parasuicidal borderline patients. Arch Gen Psychiatry 1993; 50:971–974; correction, 1994; 51:422 [A]
6. Kjelsberg E, Eikeseth PH, Dahl AA: Suicide in borderline patients—predictive factors. Acta Psychiatr Scand 1991; 84:283–287 [D]
7. Sederer LI, Ellison J, Keyes C: Guidelines for prescribing psychiatrists in consultative, collaborative, and supervisory relationships. Psychiatr Serv 1998; 49:1197–1202 [F]
8. Linehan MM, Armstrong HE, Suarez A, Allmon D, Heard HL: Cognitive-behavioral treatment of chronically parasuicidal borderline patients. Arch Gen Psychiatry 1991; 48:1060–1064 [A]
9. Bateman A, Fonagy P: Effectiveness of partial hospitalization in the treatment of borderline personality disorder: a randomized controlled trial. Am J Psychiatry 1999; 156:1563–1569 [A]
10. Bateman A, Fonagy P: Treatment of borderline personality disorder with psychoanalytically oriented partial hospitalization: an 18-month follow-up. Am J Psychiatry 2001; 158:36–42 [A]

11. Gabbard GO, Horwitz L, Allen JG, Frieswyk S, Newsom G, Colson DB, Coyne L: Transference interpretation in the psychotherapy of borderline patients: a high-risk, high-gain phenomenon. Harv Rev Psychiatry 1994; 2:59–69 [B]

12. Gunderson JG: Borderline Personality Disorder: A Clinical Guide. Washington, DC, American Psychiatric Press, 2001 [G]

13. Clarkin JF, Yeomans FE, Kernberg OF: Psychotherapy for Borderline Personality. New York, John Wiley & Sons, 1999 [G]

14. Adler G: Borderline Psychopathology and Its Treatment. New York, Jason Aronson, 1985 [G]

15. Gabbard GO, Wilkinson SM: Management of Countertransference With Borderline Patients. Washington, DC, American Psychiatric Press, 1994 [G]

16. Horwitz L, Gabbard GO, Allen JG: Borderline Personality Disorder: Tailoring the Psychotherapy to the Patient. Washington, DC, American Psychiatric Press, 1996 [B]

17. Linehan MM: Cognitive-Behavioral Treatment of Borderline Personality Disorder. New York, Guilford Press, 1993 [G]

18. Waldinger RJ: Intensive psychodynamic therapy with borderline patients: an overview. Am J Psychiatry 1987; 144:267–274 [G]

19. Beck AT, Freeman AM: Cognitive Therapy of Personality Disorders. New York, Guilford Press, 1990 [G]

20. Stevenson J, Meares R: An outcome study of psychotherapy for patients with borderline personality disorder. Am J Psychiatry 1992; 149:358–362 [B]

21. Meares R, Stevenson J, Comerford A: Psychotherapy with borderline patients, I: a comparison between treated and untreated cohorts. Aust N Z J Psychiatry 1999; 33:467–472 [B]

22. Boyer LB: Working with a borderline patient. Psychoanal Q 1977; 46:386–424 [G]

23. Chessick RD: Intensive Psychotherapy of the Borderline Patient. New York, Jason Aronson, 1977 [G]

24. Grotstein JS: The analysis of a borderline patient, in Technical Factors in the Treatment of the Severely Disturbed Patient. Edited by Giovacchini PL, Boyer LB. New York, Jason Aronson, 1982, pp 261–288 [G]

25. Grotstein JS, Solomon MF, Lang JA: The Borderline Patient: Emerging Concepts in Diagnosis, Psychodynamics, and Treatment. Hillsdale, NJ, Analytic Press, 1987 [G]

26. Gunderson JG: Borderline Personality Disorder. Washington, DC, American Psychiatric Press, 1984

27. Kernberg OF: Borderline Conditions and Pathological Narcissism. New York, Jason Aronson, 1975 [G]

28. Kernberg OF: Severe Personality Disorders: Psychotherapeutic Strategies. New Haven, Conn, Yale University Press, 1984 [G]

29. Masterson JF: Psychotherapy of the Borderline Adult: A Developmental Approach. New York, Brunner/Mazel, 1976 [G]

30. Masterson JF: The Personality Disorders: A New Look at the Developmental Self and Object Relations Approach. Phoenix, Ariz, Zeig, Tucker, 2000 [G]

31. Meares R: Metaphor of Play: Disruption and Restoration in the Borderline Experience. Northvale, NJ, Jason Aronson, 1993 [G]

32. Meares R: Intimacy and Alienation: Memory, Trauma, and Personal Being. New York, Routledge, 2000 [G]

33. Meissner WW: The Borderline Spectrum: Differential Diagnosis and Developmental Issues. New York, Jason Aronson, 1984 [G]

34. Meissner WW: Treatment of Patients in the Borderline Spectrum. Northvale, NJ, Jason Aronson, 1988 [G]

35. Rinsley DB: Developmental Pathogenesis and Treatment of Borderline and Narcissistic Personalities. Northvale, NJ, Jason Aronson, 1989 [G]

36. Searles HF: My Work With Borderline Patients. Northvale, NJ, Jason Aronson, 1986 [G]

37. Stone MH: The Borderline Syndromes: Constitution, Personality, and Adaptation. New York, McGraw-Hill, 1980 [G]

38. Waldinger RJ, Gunderson JG: Effective Psychotherapy With Borderline Patients: Case Studies. Washington, DC, American Psychiatric Press, 1987 [D]

39. Abend SM, Porder MS, Willick MS: Borderline Patients: Psychoanalytic Perspectives. Madison, Conn, International Universities Press, 1983 [G]

40. McGlashan TH: The Chestnut Lodge follow-up study, III: long-term outcome of borderline personalities. Arch Gen Psychiatry 1986; 43:20–30 [C]

41. Seeman M, Edwardes-Evans B: Marital therapy with borderline patients: is it beneficial? J Clin Psychiatry 1979; 40:308–312 [G]

42. Shapiro ER: Family dynamics and borderline personality disorder, in Handbook of Borderline Disorders. Edited by Silver D, Rosenbluth M. Madison, Conn, International Universities Press, 1992, pp 471–493 [G]

43. Siever LJ, Trestman R: The serotonin system and aggressive personality disorder. Int Clin Psychopharmacol 1993; 8:33–39 [F]

44. Salzman C, Wolfson AN, Schatzberg A, Looper J, Henke R, Albanese M, Schwartz J, Miyawaki E: Effect of fluoxetine on anger in symptomatic volunteers with borderline personality disorder. J Clin Psychopharmacol 1995; 15:23–29 [A]

45. Markovitz P: Pharmacotherapy of impulsivity, aggression, and related disorders, in Impulsivity and Aggression. Edited by Hollander E, Stein DJ. New York, John Wiley & Sons, 1995, pp 263–287 [B]

46. Cornelius JR, Soloff PH, Perel JM, Ulrich RF: Fluoxetine trial in borderline personality disorder. Psychopharmacol Bull 1990; 26:151–154 [B]

47. Kavoussi RJ, Liu J, Coccaro EF: An open trial of sertraline in personality disordered patients with impulsive aggression. J Clin Psychiatry 1994; 55:137–141 [B]

48. Markovitz PJ, Calabrese JR, Charles SC, Meltzer HY: Fluoxetine in the treatment of borderline and schizotypal personality disorders. Am J Psychiatry 1991; 148:1064–1067 [B]

49. Norden MJ: Fluoxetine in borderline personality disorder. Prog Neuropsychopharmacol Biol Psychiatry 1989; 13:885–893 [G]

50. Soloff PH, George A, Nathan RS, Schulz PM, Ulrich RF, Perel JM: Progress in pharmacotherapy of borderline disorders: a double-blind study of amitriptyline, haloperidol, and placebo. Arch Gen Psychiatry 1986; 43:691–697 [A]

51. Soloff PH, George A, Nathan S, Schulz PM, Cornelius JR, Herring J, Perel JM: Amitriptyline versus haloperidol in borderlines: final outcomes and predictors of response. J Clin Psychopharmacol 1989; 9:238–246 [A]

52. Faltus FJ: The positive effect of alprazolam in the treatment of three patients with borderline personality disorder. Am J Psychiatry 1984; 141:802–803 [G]

53. Gardner DL, Cowdry RW: Alprazolam-induced dyscontrol in borderline personality disorder. Am J Psychiatry 1985; 142:98–100 [A]

54. Freinhar JP, Alvarez WA: Clonazepam: a novel therapeutic adjunct. Int J Psychiatry Med 1985; 15:321–328 [G]

55. Cowdry RW, Gardner DL: Pharmacotherapy of borderline personality disorder: alprazolam, carbamazepine, trifluoperazine, and tranylcypromine. Arch Gen Psychiatry 1988; 45:111–119 [A]

56. Soloff PH, Cornelius J, George A, Nathan S, Perel JM, Ulrich RF: Efficacy of phenelzine and haloperidol in borderline personality disorder. Arch Gen Psychiatry 1993; 50:377–385 [A]

57. Parsons B, Quitkin FM, McGrath PJ, Stewart JW, Tricamo E, Ocepek-Welikson K, Harrison W, Rabkin JG, Wager SG, Nunes E: Phenelzine, imipramine, and placebo in borderline patients meeting criteria for atypical depression. Psychopharmacol Bull 1989; 25:524–534 [A]

58. Sheard MH: Lithium in the treatment of aggression. J Nerv Ment Dis 1975; 160:108–118 [B]

59. Sheard MH, Marini JL, Bridges CI, Wagner E: The effect of lithium on impulsive aggressive behavior in man. Am J Psychiatry 1976; 133:1409–1413 [A]

60. Tupin JP, Smith DB, Clanon TL, Kim LI, Nugent A, Groupe A: The long-term use of lithium in aggressive prisoners. Compr Psychiatry 1973; 14:311–317 [B]

61. Links P, Steiner M, Boiago I, Irwin D: Lithium therapy for borderline patients: preliminary findings. J Personal Disord 1990; 4:173–181 [A]

62. Gardner DL, Cowdry RW: Positive effects of carbamazepine on behavioral dyscontrol in borderline personality disorder. Am J Psychiatry 1986; 143:519–522 [A]

63. De la Fuente J, Lotstra F: A trial of carbamazepine in borderline personality disorder. Eur Neuropsychopharmacol 1994; 4:479–486 [A]

64. Gardner DL, Cowdry RW: Development of melancholia during carbamazepine treatment in borderline personality disorder. J Clin Psychopharmacol 1986; 6:236–239 [A]

65. Hollander E, Allen A, Lopez RP, Bienstock C, Grossman R, Siever L, Margolin L, Stein D: A preliminary double-blind, placebo-controlled trial of divalproex sodium in borderline personality disorder. J Clin Psychiatry 2001; 62:199–203 [A]

66. Stein DJ, Simeon D, Frenkel M, Islam MN, Hollander E: An open trial of valproate in borderline personality disorder. J Clin Psychiatry 1995; 56:506–510 [B]

67. Coccaro EF, Kavoussi RJ: Fluoxetine and impulsive aggressive behavior in personality-disordered subjects. Arch Gen Psychiatry 1997; 54:1081–1088 [A]

68. Cornelius JR, Soloff PH, Perel JM, Ulrich RF: Continuation pharmacotherapy of borderline personality disorder with haloperidol and phenelzine. Am J Psychiatry 1993; 150:1843–1848 [A]

69. Kavoussi RJ, Coccaro EF: Divalproex sodium for impulsive aggressive behavior in patients with personality disorder. J Clin Psychiatry 1998; 59:676–680 [B]

70. Wilcox J: Divalproex sodium in the treatment of aggressive behavior. Ann Clin Psychiatry 1994; 6:17–20 [B]

71. Benedetti F, Sforzini L, Colombo C, Maffei C, Smeraldi E: Low-dose clozapine in acute and continuation treatment of severe borderline personality disorder. J Clin Psychiatry 1998; 59:103–107 [B]

72. Chengappa KN, Baker RW: The successful use of clozapine in ameliorating severe self mutilation in a patient with borderline personality disorder. J Personal Disord 1995; 9: 76–82 [G]

73. Leone N: Response of borderline patients to loxapine and chlorpromazine. J Clin Psychiatry 1982; 43:148–150 [A]

74. Serban G, Siegel S: Response of borderline and schizotypal patients to small doses of thiothixene and haloperidol. Am J Psychiatry 1984; 141:1455–1458 [A]

75. Goldberg S, Schulz C, Schulz P, Resnick R, Hamer R, Friedel R: Borderline and schizotypal personality disorder treated with low-dose thiothixene vs placebo. Arch Gen Psychiatry 1986; 43:680–686 [A]

76. Goldberg S: Prediction of change in borderline personality disorder. Psychopharmacol Bull 1989; 25:550–555 [E]

77. Kutcher S, Papatheodorou G, Reiter S, Gardner D: The successful pharmacological treatment of adolescents and young adults with borderline personality disorder: a preliminary open trial of flupenthixol. J Psychiatry Neurosci 1995; 20:113–118 [B]

78. Teicher M, Glod C, Aaronson S, Gunter P, Schatzberg A, Cole J: Open assessment of the safety and efficacy of thioridazine in the treatment of patients with borderline personality disorder. Psychopharmacol Bull 1989; 25:535–549 [B]

79. Kelly T, Soloff PH, Cornelius JR, George A, Lis J: Can we study (treat) borderline patients: attrition from research and open treatment. J Personal Disord 1992; 6:417–433 [A]

80. Montgomery SA, Montgomery D: Pharmacological prevention of suicidal behaviour. J Affect Disord 1982; 4:291–298 [A]

81. Frankenburg F, Zanarini MC: Clozapine treatment of borderline patients: a preliminary study. Compr Psychiatry 1993; 34:402–405 [B]

82. Schulz S, Camlin KL, Berry SA, Jesberger JA: Olanzapine safety and efficacy in patients with borderline personality disorder and comorbid dysthymia. Biol Psychiatry 1999; 46: 1429–1435 [B]

83. Schulz SC, Camlin KL, Berry S, Friedman L: Risperidone for borderline personality disorder: a double blind study, in Proceedings of the 39th Annual Meeting of the American College of Neuropsychopharmacology. Nashville, Tenn, ACNP, 1999 [A]

84. American Psychiatric Association: Practice Guideline for the Treatment of Patients With Major Depressive Disorder (Revision). Am J Psychiatry 2000; 157(April suppl) [G]

85. American Psychiatric Association: Practice Guideline for the Treatment of Patients With Bipolar Disorder. Am J Psychiatry 1994; 151(Dec suppl) [G]

86. American Psychiatric Association: Practice Guideline for the Treatment of Patients With Eating Disorders (Revision). Am J Psychiatry 2000; 157(Jan suppl) [G]

87. American Psychiatric Association: Practice Guideline for the Treatment of Patients With Substance Use Disorders: Alcohol, Cocaine, Opioids. Am J Psychiatry 1995; 152(Nov suppl) [G]

88. American Psychiatric Association: Practice Guideline for the Treatment of Patients With Panic Disorder. Am J Psychiatry 1998; 155(May suppl) [G]

89. Soloff P, Cornelius J, George A: Relationship between axis I and axis II disorders: implications for treatment. Psychopharmacol Bull 1991; 27:23–30 [F]

90. Soloff PH, George A, Nathan RS, Schulz PM: Characterizing depression in borderline patients. J Clin Psychiatry 1987; 48:155–157 [E]

91. Rogers JH, Widiger TA, Krupp A: Aspects of depression associated with borderline personality disorder. Am J Psychiatry 1995; 152:268–270 [D]

92. Gunderson JG, Phillips KA: A current view of the interface between borderline personality disorder and depression. Am J Psychiatry 1991; 148:967–975 [F]

93. Stone MH: Abnormalities of Personality: Within and Beyond the Realm of Treatment. New York, WW Norton, 1993 [G]

94. Losel F: Management of psychopaths, in Psychopathy: Theory, Research and Implications for Society. Edited by Cooke DJ, Forth AE, Hare RD. Boston, Kluwer, 1998, pp 303–354 [G]

95. Dolan BM, Evans C, Wilson J: Therapeutic community treatment for personality disordered adults: changes in neurotic symptomatology on follow-up. Int J Soc Psychiatry 1992; 38:243–250 [B]

96. Coccaro EF, Kavoussi RJ, Sheline YI, Lish JD, Csernansky JG: Impulsive aggression in personality disorder correlates with tritiated paroxetine binding in the platelet. Arch Gen Psychiatry 1996; 53:531–536 [G]

97. Hare RD: The Hare Psychopathy Checklist—Revised. North Tonawanda, NY, Mental Health Systems, 1991 [G]

98. Gunderson JG, Sabo AN: The phenomenological and conceptual interface between borderline personality disorder and PTSD. Am J Psychiatry 1993; 150:19–27 [F]

99. Gunderson JG, Chu JA: Treatment implications of past trauma in borderline personality disorder. Harv Rev Psychiatry 1993; 1:75–81 [F]

100. Paris J, Zweig-Frank H: Dissociation in patients with borderline personality disorder (letter). Am J Psychiatry 1997; 154:137–138 [F]

101. Resnick HS, Kilpatrick DG, Dansky BS, Saunders BE, Best CL: Prevalence of civilian trauma and posttraumatic stress disorder in a representative national sample of women. J Consult Clin Psychol 1993; 61:984–991 [D]

102. Davidson JR, Hughes D, Blazer DG, George LK: Post-traumatic stress disorder in the community: an epidemiological study. Psychol Med 1991; 21:713–721 [D]

103. Ogata SN, Silk KR, Goodrich S, Lohr NE, Westen D, Hill EM: Childhood sexual and physical abuse in adult patients with borderline personality disorder. Am J Psychiatry 1990; 147:1008–1013 [D]

104. Fossati A, Madeddu F, Maffei C: Borderline personality disorder and childhood sexual abuse: a meta-analytic study. J Personal Disord 1999; 13:268–280 [E]

105. Lindemann E: Symptomatology and management of acute grief (1944). Am J Psychiatry 1994; 151(June suppl):155–160 [G]

106. Spiegel D: Vietnam grief work using hypnosis. Am J Clin Hypn 1981; 24:33–40 [B]

107. Butler LD, Duran REF, Jasiukaitis P, Kopan C, Spiegel D: Hypnotizability and traumatic experience: a diathesis-stress model of dissociative symptomatology (festschrift). Am J Psychiatry 1996; 153(July suppl):42–63 [F]

108. Shapiro F: Eye movement desensitization and reprocessing (EMDR) and the anxiety disorders: clinical and research implications of an integrated psychotherapy treatment. J Anxiety Disord 1999; 13:35–67 [F]

109. Wilson SA, Becker LA, Tinker RH: Eye movement desensitization and reprocessing (EMDR) treatment for psychologically traumatized individuals. J Consult Clin Psychol 1995; 63:928–937 [A]

110. Wilson SA, Becker LA, Tinker RH: Fifteen-month follow-up of eye movement desensitization and reprocessing (EMDR) treatment for posttraumatic stress disorder and psychological trauma. J Consult Clin Psychol 1997; 65:1047–1056 [B]

111. Jones B, Heard H, Startup M, Swales M, Williams JM, Jones RS: Autobiographical memory and dissociation in borderline personality disorder. Psychol Med 1999; 29:1397–1404 [D]

112. Chu JA, Dill DL: Dissociative symptoms in relation to childhood physical and sexual abuse. Am J Psychiatry 1990; 147:887–892 [D]

113. Neisser U, Fivush R (eds): The Remembering Self: Construction and Accuracy in the Self-Narrative. New York, Cambridge University Press, 1994 [G]

114. Saxe GN, van der Kolk BA, Berkowitz R, Chinman G, Hall K, Lieberg G, Schwartz J: Dissociative disorders in psychiatric inpatients. Am J Psychiatry 1993; 150:1037–1042 [D]

115. Galletly C: Borderline-dissociation comorbidity (letter). Am J Psychiatry 1997; 154:1629 [G]

116. Brodsky BS, Cloitre M, Dulit RA: Relationship of dissociation to self-mutilation and childhood abuse in borderline personality disorder. Am J Psychiatry 1995; 152:1788–1792 [D]

117. Ross CA, Miller SD, Reagor P, Bjornson L, Fraser GA, Anderson G: Structured interview data on 102 cases of multiple personality disorder from four centers. Am J Psychiatry 1990; 147:596–601 [D]

118. Braun BG, Sacks RG: The development of multiple personality disorder: predisposing, precipitating, and perpetuating factors, in Childhood Antecedents of Multiple Personality. Edited by Kluft RP. Washington, DC, American Psychiatric Press, 1985, pp 37–64 [F]

119. Kluft RP: The use of hypnosis with dissociative disorders. Psychiatr Med 1992; 10:31–46 [F]

120. Spiegel D, Maldonado J: Dissociative disorders, in The American Psychiatric Press Textbook of Psychiatry, 3rd ed. Edited by Hales RE, Yudofsky S, Talbott JA. Washington, DC, American Psychiatric Press, 1999, pp 711–737 [F]

121. Spiegel D: Dissociative Disorders: A Clinical Review. Lutherville, Md, Sidran Press, 1996, pp 1156–1172 [G]

122. Paris J, Zelkowitz P, Guzder J, Joseph S, Feldman R: Neuropsychological factors associated with borderline pathology in children. J Am Acad Child Adolesc Psychiatry 1999; 38:770–774 [D]

123. Zanarini MC, Williams AA, Lewis RE, Reich RB, Vera SC, Marino MF, Levin A, Yong L, Frankenburg FR: Reported pathological childhood experiences associated with the development of borderline personality disorder. Am J Psychiatry 1997; 154:1101–1106 [D]

124. Paris J: The etiology of borderline personality disorder: a biopsychosocial approach. Psychiatry 1994; 57:316–325 [F]

125. Altshuler LL, Cohen L, Szuba MP, Burt VK, Gitlin M, Mintz J: Pharmacologic management of psychiatric illness during pregnancy: dilemmas and guidelines. Am J Psychiatry 1996; 153:592–606 [F]

126. Cohen LS, Heller VL, Rosenbaum JF: Treatment guidelines for psychotropic drug use in pregnancy. Psychosomatics 1989; 30:25–33 [G]

127. Cohen L: Approach to the patient with psychiatric disorders during pregnancy, in The MGH Guide to Psychiatry and Primary Care. New York, McGraw-Hill, 1998, pp 311–317 [F]

128. Omtzigt JG, Los FJ, Grobbee DE, Pijpers L, Jahoda MG, Brandenburg H, Stewart PA, Gaillard HL, Sachs ES, Wladimiroff JW: The risk of spina bifida aperta after first-trimester exposure to valproate in a prenatal cohort. Neurology 1992; 42:119–125 [G]

129. Loranger AW, Sartorius N, Andreoli A, Berger P, Buchheim P, Channabasavanna SM, Coid B, Dahl A, Diekstra RFW, Ferguson B, Jacobsberg LB, Mombour W, Pull C, Ono Y, Regier DA: The International Personality Disorder Examination: the World Health Organization/Alcohol, Drug Abuse, and Mental Health Administration International Pilot Study of Personality Disorders. Arch Gen Psychiatry 1994; 51:215–224 [B]

130. Kissling W (ed): Guidelines for Neuroleptic Relapse Prevention in Schizophrenia. Berlin, Springer-Verlag, 1991 [G]

131. Marcos LR, Cancro R: Pharmacotherapy of Hispanic depressed patients: clinical observations. Am J Psychother 1982; 36:505–512 [F]

132. Escobar JI, Tuason VB: Antidepressant agents: a cross-cultural study. Psychopharmacol Bull 1980; 16:49–52 [F]

133. Klein JI, Macbeth JE, Onek JN: Legal Issues in the Private Practice of Psychiatry. Washington, DC, American Psychiatric Press, 1994 [G]

134. Paris J, Brown R, Nowlis D: Long-term follow-up of borderline patients in a general hospital. Compr Psychiatry 1987; 28:530–535 [D]

135. Bender DS, Dolan RT, Skodol AE, Sanislow CA, Dyck IR, McGlashan TH, Shea MT, Zanarini MC, Oldham JM, Gunderson JG: Treatment utilization by patients with personality disorders. Am J Psychiatry 2001; 158:295–302 [C]

136. Phillips KA, Gunderson JG: Personality disorders, in The American Psychiatric Press Textbook of Psychiatry, 3rd ed. Edited by Hales RE, Yudofsky SC, Talbott JA. Washington, DC, American Psychiatric Press, 1999, pp 795–823 [G]

137. Stone MH: Long-Term Follow-Up Study of Borderline Patients: The Fate of Borderlines. New York, Guilford, 1990 [C]

138. Stevenson J, Meares R: Psychotherapy with borderline patients, II: a preliminary cost benefit study. Aust N Z J Psychiatry 1999; 33:473–477 [B]

139. Gabbard GO: Psychodynamic Psychiatry in Clinical Practice, 3rd ed. Washington, DC, American Psychiatric Press, 2000 [G]

140. Clarkin JF, Yeomans F, Kernberg OF: Psychodynamic Psychotherapy of Borderline Personality Organization: A Treatment Manual. New York, John Wiley & Sons, 1998 [G]

141. Wallerstein RW: Forty-Two Lives in Treatment. New York, Guilford, 1986 [D]

142. Howard KI, Kopta SM, Krause MS, Orlinsky DE: The dose-effect relationship in psychotherapy. Am Psychol 1986; 41:159–164 [D]

143. Gabbard GO: Borderline Personality Disorder and Rational Managed Care Policy. Psychoanal Inquiry Suppl 1997, pp 17–28 [G]

144. Beck JS: Complex cognitive therapy treatment for personality disorder patients. Bull Menninger Clin 1998; 62:170–194 [G]

145. Layden MA, Newman CF, Freeman A, Morse SB: Cognitive Therapy of Borderline Personality Disorder. Boston, Allyn & Bacon, 1993 [G]

146. Millon T: On the genesis and prevalence of the borderline personality disorder: a social learning thesis. J Personal Disord 1987; 1:354–372 [G]

147. Young JE: Cognitive Therapy for Personality Disorders: A Schema-Focused Approach. Sarasota, Fla, Professional Resource Exchange, 1990 [G]

148. Linehan MM, Tutek DA, Heard HL, Armstrong HE: Interpersonal outcome of cognitive behavioral treatment for chronically suicidal borderline patients. Am J Psychiatry 1994; 151:1771–1776 [B]

149. Linehan MM, Schmidt H III, Dimeff LA, Craft JC, Kanter J, Comtois KA: Dialectical behavior therapy for patients with borderline personality disorder and drug-dependence. Am J Addict 1999; 8:279–292 [A]

150. Linehan MM, Heard HL: Impact of treatment accessibility on clinical course of para-suicidal patients (letter). Arch Gen Psychiatry 1993; 50:157–158 [G]

151. Springer T, Lohr NE, Buchtel HA, Silk KR: A preliminary report of short-term cognitive-behavioral group therapy for inpatients with personality disorders. J Psychother Pract Res 1995; 5:57–71 [A]

152. Barley W, Buie SE, Peterson EW, Hollingsworth A, Griva M, Hickerson S, Lawson J, Bailey B: Development of an inpatient cognitive-behavioral treatment program for borderline personality disorder. J Personal Disord 1993; 7:232–240 [B]

153. Perris C: Cognitive therapy in the treatment of patients with borderline personality disorders. Acta Psychiatr Scand Suppl 1994; 379:69–72 [F]

154. Liberman RP, Eckman T: Behavior therapy vs insight-oriented therapy for repeated suicide attempters. Arch Gen Psychiatry 1981; 38:1126–1130 [A]

155. Salkovskis PM, Atha C, Storer D: Cognitive-behavioural problem solving in the treatment of patients who repeatedly attempt suicide: a controlled trial. Br J Psychiatry 1990; 157:871–876 [A]

156. Evans K, Tyrer P, Catalan J, Schmidt U, Davidson K, Dent J, Tata P, Thornton S, Barber J, Thompson S: Manual-assisted cognitive-behaviour therapy (MACT): a randomized controlled trial of a brief intervention with bibliotherapy in the treatment of recurrent deliberate self-harm. Psychol Med 1999; 29:19–25 [A]

157. Greene LR, Cole MB: Level and form of psychopathology and the structure of group therapy. Int J Group Psychother 1991; 41:499–521 [B]

158. Hafner RJ, Holme G: The influence of a therapeutic community on psychiatric disorder. J Clin Psychol 1996; 52:461–468 [C]

159. Goodwin JM, Wilson N, Connell V: Natural history of severe symptoms in borderline women treated in an incest group. Dissociation 1994; 5:221–226 [D]

160. Marziali E, Munroe-Blum H, McCleary L: The contribution of group cohesion and group alliance to the outcome of group psychotherapy. Int J Group Psychother 1997; 47:475–497 [A]

161. Wilberg T, Friis S, Karterud S, Mehlum L, Urnes O, Vaglum P: Outpatient group psychotherapy: a valuable continuation treatment for patients with borderline personality disorder treated in a day hospital? a 3-year follow-up study. Nord Psykiatr Tidsskr 1998; 52:213–222 [B]

162. Higgitt A, Fonagy P: Psychotherapy in borderline and narcissistic personality disorder. Br J Psychiatry 1992; 161:23–43 [F]

163. Marziali E, Monroe-Blum H: Interpersonal Group Psychotherapy for Borderline Personality Disorder. New York, Basic Books, 1994 [A]

164. Koch A, Ingram T: The treatment of borderline personality disorder within a distressed relationship. J Marital Fam Ther 1985; 11:373–380 [G]

165. Weddige R: The hidden psychotherapeutic dilemma: spouse of the borderline. Am J Psychother 1986; 40:52–61 [G]

166. McCormack C: The borderline/schizoid marriage: the holding environment as an essential treatment construct. J Marital Fam Ther 1989; 15:299–309 [G]

167. Jones SA: Family therapy with borderline and narcissistic patients. Bull Menninger Clin 1987; 51:285–295 [G]

168. Clarkin JF, Marziali E, Munroe-Blum H: Group and family treatments for borderline personality disorder. Hosp Community Psychiatry 1991; 42:1038–1043 [F]

169. Villeneuve C, Roux N: Family therapy and some personality disorders in adolescence. Adolesc Psychiatry 1995; 20:365–380 [G]

170. Gunderson JG, Berkowitz C, Ruiz-Sancho A: Families of borderline patients: a psycho-educational approach. Bull Menninger Clin 1997; 61:446–457 [G]

171. Gunderson JG, Kerr J, Englund DW: The families of borderlines: a comparative study. Arch Gen Psychiatry 1980; 37:27–33 [D]

172. Markovitz P, Wagner S: Venlafaxine in the treatment of borderline personality disorder. Psychopharmacol Bull 1995; 31:773–777 [B]

173. Coccaro EF, Astill JL, Herbert JL, Schut AG: Fluoxetine treatment of impulsive aggression in DSM-III-R personality disorder patients (letter). J Clin Psychopharmacol 1990; 10:373–375 [G]

174. Jensen HV, Andersen J: An open, noncomparative study of amoxapine in borderline disorders. Acta Psychiatr Scand 1989; 79:89–93 [B]

175. Montgomery SA, Roy D, Montgomery DB: The prevention of recurrent suicidal acts. Br J Clin Pharmacol 1983; 15(suppl 2):183S–188S [A]

176. Pande AC, Birkett M, Fechner-Bates S, Haskett RF, Greden JF: Fluoxetine versus phenelzine in atypical depression. Biol Psychiatry 1996; 40:1017–1020 [A]

177. Soloff PH, George A, Nathan RS, Schulz PM, Perel JM: Behavioral dyscontrol in borderline patients treated with amitriptyline. Psychopharmacol Bull 1987; 23:177–181 [A]

178. Shader RI, DiMascio A: Psychotropic Drug Side Effects. Baltimore, Williams and Wilkins, 1970 [G]

179. Rifkin A, Levitan SJ, Galewski J, Klein DF: Emotionally unstable character disorder—a follow-up study, I: description of patients and outcome. Biol Psychiatry 1972; 4:65–79 [C]

180. Rifkin A, Levitan SJ, Galewski J, Klein DF: Emotionally unstable character disorder—a follow-up study, II: prediction of outcome. Biol Psychiatry 1972; 4:81–88 [C]

181. Shader RI, Jackson AH, Dodes LM: The antiaggressive effects of lithium in man. Psychopharmacologia 1974; 40:17–24 [G]

182. LaWall JS, Wesselius CL: The use of lithium carbonate in borderline patients. J Psychiatr Treatment and Evaluation 1982; 4:265–267 [G]

183. Pinto OC, Akiskal HS: Lamotrigine as a promising approach to borderline personality: an open case series without concurrent DSM-IV major mood disorder. J Affect Disord 1998; 51:333–343 [B]

184. Wolf M, Grayden T, Carreon D, Cosgro M, Summers D, Leino R, Goldstein J, Kim S: Psychotherapy and buspirone in borderline patients, in 1990 Annual Meeting New Research Program and Abstracts. Washington, DC, American Psychiatric Association, 1990, p 244 [B]

185. Winchel RM, Stanley M: Self-injurious behavior: a review of the behavior and biology of self-mutilation. Am J Psychiatry 1991; 148:306–317 [F]

186. van der Kolk BA, Greenberg MS, Orr SP, Pitman RK: Endogenous opioids, stress induced analgesia, and posttraumatic stress disorder. Psychopharmacol Bull 1989; 25:417–421 [F]

187. Konicki PE, Schulz SC: Rationale for clinical trials of opiate antagonists in treating patients with personality disorders and self-injurious behavior. Psychopharmacol Bull 1989; 25:556–563 [E]

188. McGee M: Cessation of self-mutilation in a patient with borderline personality disorder treated with naltrexone. J Clin Psychiatry 1997; 58:32–33 [E]

189. Sonne S, Rubey R, Brady K, Malcolm R, Morris T: Naltrexone treatment of self-injurious thoughts and behaviors. J Nerv Ment Dis 1996; 184:192–195 [B]

190. Roth AS, Ostroff RB, Hoffman RE: Naltrexone as a treatment for repetitive self-injurious behaviour: an open-label trial. J Clin Psychiatry 1996; 57:233–237 [B]

191. Russ M, Roth SD, Kakuma T, Harrison K, Hull JW: Pain perception in self-injurious borderline patients: naloxone effects. Biol Psychiatry 1994; 35:207–209 [B]

192. Black DW, Bell S, Hulbert J, Nasrallah A: The importance of axis II in patients with major depression: a controlled study. J Affect Disord 1988; 14:115–122 [D]

193. Black DW, Goldstein RB, Nasrallah A, Winokur G: The prediction of recovery using a multivariate model in 1471 depressed inpatients. Eur Arch Psychiatry Clin Neurosci 1991; 241:41–45 [E]

194. Zimmerman M, Coryell W, Pfohl B, Corenthal C, Stangl D: ECT response in depressed patients with and without a DSM-III personality disorder. Am J Psychiatry 1986; 143: 1030–1032 [B]

195. Pfohl B, Stangl D, Zimmerman M: The implications of DSM-III personality disorders for patients with major depression. J Affect Disord 1984; 7:309–318 [B]

196. Casey P, Butler E: The effects of personality on response to ECT in major depression. J Personal Disord 1995; 9:134–142 [B]

197. Casey P, Meagher D, Butler E: Personality, functioning, and recovery from major depression. J Nerv Ment Dis 1996; 184:240–245 [B]

198. Blais MA, Matthews J, Schouten R, O'Keefe SM, Summergrad P: Stability and predictive value of self-report personality traits pre- and post-electroconvulsive therapy: a preliminary study. Compr Psychiatry 1998; 39:231–235 [B]